Revision for the MRCPsych

CW00518748

Revision for the MRCPsych Part I

B. K. Puri
MA MB BChir MRCPsych
Senior Registrar in Psychiatry,
Charing Cross and Westminster Hospitals, London

J. Sklar
LRCP MRCS MB BS MRCPsych AssMemBritPsychoanalSoc
Psychoanalyst and Consultant Psychotherapist,
Department of Psychotherapy,
Addenbrooke's and Fulbourn Hospitals, Cambridge

Foreword by

Professor S. R. Hirsch
BA MD MPhil FRCP FRCPsych
Professor of Psychiatry and Honorary Consultant,
Department of Psychiatry,
Charing Cross and Westminster Medical School, London

Churchill Livingstone

EDINBURGH LONDON MELBOURNE AND NEW YORK 1990

CHURCHILL LIVINGSTONE
Medical Division of Longman Group UK Limited

Distributed in the United States of America by
Churchill Livingstone Inc., 1560 Broadway, New
York, N.Y. 10036, and by associated companies,
branches and representatives throughout the
world.

First published 1990

ISBN 0-443-04331-0

British Library Cataloguing in Publication Data
Puri, B. K.
    Revision for the MRCPsych part I.
    1. Medicine. Psychiatry
    I. Title II. Sklar, J.
    616.89

Library of Congress Cataloging in Publication Data
Puri, Basant K.
    Revision for the MRCPsych part I /B. K. Puri,
    J. Sklar; foreword by S.R. Hirsch.
        p. cm.
    ISBN 0-443-04331-0
    1. Psychiatry — Examinations, questions,
etc. 2. Neurology — Examinations,
questions, etc. I. Sklar, J.
(Jonathan) II. Title.
    [DNLM: 1. Psychiatry — examination
questions. WM 18 P985r]
RC457.P8695   1990
616.89'0076 — dc20
DNLM/DLC
for Library of Congress   89-71314

Produced by Longman Singapore Publishers (Pte) Ltd.
Printed in Singapore.

Foreword

While students and doctors in training often feel that examinations are an unwanted burden, most of us agree that they motivate learning and 'focus the mind wonderfully'. If this is so, then having completed the phase when information is assimilated, the objectives of focusing attention and stimulating learning should be abetted by an opportunity to test one's knowledge and ability, and find weak spots which can be rectified. An opportunity to practise the examination itself so that the candidate can become experienced in the form and procedure of the examination while using questions which cover the subject matter they are likely to encounter, helps to eliminate distractions and erroneous misunderstandings which could otherwise distract from the candidate's concentration and performance. Thus the concept of a practice examination with real life questions and answers should contribute to the learning process, improve candidates' performance and improve the validity of the examination result.

This straightforward book of sample multiple choice questions for the Part I for the MRCPsych provides the stimulus that students need as they come into the final stages of preparation and learning. Each section of the book covers a different aspect of the MRCPsych Part I examination and describes what the syllabus requires for that section. Neuroanatomy and physiology, basic pharmacology, general and dynamic psychopathology, clinical assessment, and classification are all covered. The subject is broadly and accurately dealt with and the answers to questions are exceptionally clear and helpful. Students should work through each section quickly, answering all the questions and then check their performance. After that they should consult the correct response to check their reasoning and explain incorrect responses. I recommend this as an excellent revision for the MRCPsych Part I.

Steven R. Hirsch

Preface

The MRCPsych Part I examination consists of one multiple choice paper of 50 questions, and a clinical examination. The latter must be passed in order to pass overall. The authors are of the view that the best preparation for the clinical part is regular practice in clerking and presenting patients. It is important also, in the authors' view, for candidates to gain experience in answering multiple choice questions and to test their theoretical knowledge. This book is aimed at helping with such preparation for the multiple choice question papers of the MRCPsych Part I and equivalent examinations. It has been designed largely as a companion to the authors' sister revision book *Examination Notes for the MRCPsych Part I*[1].

The definitions of the words used in the stems of the multiple choice questions have been based on those given by Dr J. Anderson in his excellent book *The Multiple Choice Question in Medicine*[2]. The syllabus used as the basis of the multiple choice questions is that given in the Eighth Revision of the *General Information and Regulations for the MRCPsych Examinations*[3]. The questions are based on those given in the *Working Party for Review of the MRCPsych Report to the Court of Electors*[4].

We should like to thank Georgina Bentliff and her colleagues at Churchill Livingstone for their kind help and encouragement.

We should also like to thank Professor Hirsch for kindly providing a Foreword.

Cambridge 1990   B.P.
                                                                 J.S.

1. Puri B K and Sklar J 1989 Examination Notes for the MRCPsych Part I. Butterworths, London
2. Anderson J 1982 The Multiple Choice Question in Medicine, 2nd edn. Pitman, London
3. The Royal College of Psychiatrists 1987 General Information and Regulations for the MRCPsych Examinations, 8th revision. The Royal College of Psychiatrists, London
4. The Royal College of Psychiatrists 1985 Report to the Court of Electors, The Royal College of Psychiatrists Working Party for Review of the MRCPsych. The Royal College of Psychiatrists, London

Contents

1. Neuroanatomy and neurophysiology

Syllabus requirements

In neuroanatomy the candidate's knowledge of the brain and spinal cord and peripheral nervous system should be updated as the basis of neurological examination and diagnosis.

The physiology of the motor and sensory systems and the autonomic nervous system should be understood to a similar level.

(The anatomy and physiology of the limbic system is part of the MRCPsych Part II syllabus.)

Question 1.1

Branches of the internal carotid artery include the:
A posterior inferior cerebellar artery
B anterior cerebral artery
C middle cerebral artery
D basilar artery
E posterior communicating artery.

Answer 1.1

The brain is supplied by the internal carotid and vertebral arteries, branches of which anastomose to form the circle or polygon of Willis, also known as the circulus arteriosus. The circulus arteriosus surrounds the optic chiasma, and is formed by the following arteries:

- anterior cerebral
- anterior communicating
- middle cerebral
- posterior cerebral
- posterior communicating

A   False
The posterior inferior cerebellar artery is the largest branch of the vertebral artery.

B   True
The anterior cerebral artery is the smaller of the two terminal branches of the internal carotid artery.

C   True
The middle cerebral artery is the larger of the two terminal branches of the internal carotid artery. Indeed, it is the largest branch of the latter.

D   False
The basilar artery is formed by the joining together of the right and left vertebral arteries. It gives rise to the posterior cerebral arteries.

E   True
The posterior communicating artery arises near the terminal bifurcation of the internal carotid artery.

Question 1.2

Structures supplied by the middle cerebral artery include the:

A caudate nucleus

B occipital pole

C internal capsule

D medial aspect of the cerebral hemisphere

E midbrain.

Answer 1.2

The anterior cerebral artery supplies the medial and superolateral aspect of the cerebral hemisphere, and parts of the lentiform and caudate nuclei and the internal capsule.

The middle cerebral artery supplies most of the lateral aspect of the cerebral cortex, the lentiform and caudate nuclei, and the internal capsule.

The posterior cerebral artery supplies the inferolateral aspect of the temporal lobe, the lateral and medial aspects of the occipital lobe, parts of the thalamus and lentiform nucleus, the medial geniculate bodies, the midbrain, the pineal gland, and the choroid plexuses of the lateral and third ventricles.

A   True
The caudate nucleus receives a blood supply from both the middle and anterior cerebral arteries.

B   False
The occipital pole is supplied by the posterior cerebral artery.

C   True
The internal capsule receives a blood supply from both the middle and anterior cerebral arteries.

D   False
The middle cerebral artery supplies most of the lateral aspect of the cerebral cortex.

E   False
The midbrain is supplied by the posterior cerebral artery.

Question 1.3

Types of glial cells found in the central nervous system include:

A oligodendrocytes

B Golgi cells

C tanycytes

D stellate cells

E ependymal cells.

Answer 1.3

The neuroglia are also known as interstitial cells and make up most of the nervous tissue, outnumbering neurones five to ten times. They consist of the following main types:

- astrocytes (astroglia)
- oligodendrocytes (oligodendroglia)
- microglia
- ependyma

A True
Oligodendrocytes form the myelin sheaths of central nervous system fibres. Compared with astrocytes, oligodendrocytes have a smaller perikaryon, with fewer processes.

B False
Golgi cells are found in the cerebellum and are not glial cells.

C True
Tanycytes are a form of ependyma. Tanycytes line the third ventricle floor over the hypothalamic median eminence. Other types of ependyma include:

- ependymocytes, which line the central canal of the spinal cord and the ventricles;
- choroidal epithelial cells, which cover the surfaces of the choroidal plexuses and have tight junctions.

D False
Stellate cells are found in the cerebellum and are not glial cells.

E True
Ependymal cells line the cavities of the central nervous system.

Question 1.4

Layers of the cerebral cortex include the:
A Purkinje cell layer
B polymorphic cell layer
C ganglionic layer
D molecular layer
E external granular layer.

Answer 1.4

Developmentally, the cerebral cortex consists of

(a) the archicortex or limbic formation
  — has three cellular layers
(b) the paleocortex or primary olfactory area
  — has three cellular layers
(c) the neocortex
  — makes up about 9/10 of the human cerebral cortex
  — consists of six cellular layers, as follows:

- the molecular or plexiform layer, the most superficial layer
- the external granular layer
- the external pyramidal layer
- the internal granular layer
- the ganglionic or internal pyramidal layer
- the multiform or polymorphic cell layer

A   False
The Purkinje cell layer is one of the layers of the cerebellum.

B   True
See above.

C   True
See above.

D   True
The cerebellum also has a molecular layer.

E   True
The cerebellum also has a granular layer.

Question 1.5

The following are found in the cerebellum:

A Betz cells

B Schwann cells

C basket cells

D climbing fibres

E Meissner's corpuscles.

Answer 1.5

A   False
Betz cells are giant pyramidal cells found in the primary motor area of the cerebral cortex. Whilst in other respects the premotor area, which lies anterior to the primary motor area, resembles the latter at the histological level, Betz cells are generally lacking.

B   False
Schwann cells form the myelin sheaths of peripheral nerve axons and also encircle some unmyelinated peripheral nerve axons. They are not found in the cerebellum.

C   True
The cerebellar cortex has a uniform structure in all parts of the organ and consists of three layers, the middle of which is a layer of one or two rows of large Purkinje cells associated with basket cells.

D   True
Together with mossy fibres, climbing fibres provide an excitatory input to the cells of the cerebellum. Climbing fibres represent the terminal fibres of the olivocerebellar tracts whilst mossy fibres are the terminal fibres of all the other cerebellar afferent tracts. Both types of fibre also send branches to the deep cerebellar nuclei.

E   False
Meissner's corpuscles are a form of specialized encapsulated sensory receptor or exteroceptor present in the skin. They respond to touch sensation and allow two-point tactile discrimination to occur in those areas where they are present in greater density, such as the fingers and palms.

Question 1.6

The oculomotor nerve:

A carries parasympathetic fibres

B supplies the lateral rectus muscle

C runs close to the apex of the petrous temporal bone

D is the fourth cranial nerve

E if divided results in ptosis.

Answer 1.6

The oculomotor nerve is the third cranial nerve and has two motor nuclei:

(i)   the main oculomotor nucleus;
(ii) the accessory parasympathetic or Edinger–Westphal nucleus.

The main oculomotor nucleus supplies all the extrinsic ocular muscles except the superior oblique and the lateral rectus.

Preganglionic parasympathetic fibres pass to the ciliary ganglion from whence efferent fibres pass to the ciliary muscle and the constrictor pupillae of the iris; stimulation leads to pupil constriction and lens accommodation.

A True
See above.

B False
The lateral rectus muscle is supplied by the abducent or sixth cranial nerve.

C False
The abducent nerve runs close to this bony structure. Raised intracranial pressure can cause this cranial nerve to be stretched over this structure. In addition, osteitis of the apex of the petrous temporal bone owing to otitis media can also damage it, leading to a unilateral palsy of this nerve. This is known as Gradenigo's syndrome.

D False
See above.

E True
Complete division of the third cranial nerve leads to paralysis of the levator palpebrae superioris, and hence ptosis. Other features include pupillary dilatation, constrictor pupillae paralysis (hence a loss of the light and accommodation reflexes), a divergent squint, and double vision.

Question 1.7

The olfactory nerves:

A   may be interrupted by fractures of the middle cranial fossa following head injury

B   pass through the cribriform plate of the sphenoid bone

C   are the peripheral processes of a central group of cells in the olfactory bulbs

D   carry sensory information destined for the periamygdaloid and prepiriform areas of the cerebral cortex

E   are highly likely to be damaged, following head injury, in a patient who is unaffected after attempting to smell concentrated ammonia on clinical examination.

Answer 1.7

The olfactory nerve is the first cranial nerve. Olfactory receptor central processes pass from the olfactory mucosa, superiorly through the cribriform plate of the ethmoid bone, and synapse with the olfactory bulb mitral cells. From here the mitral cell axons pass in the olfactory tract, via the lateral olfactory striae, to the periamygdaloid and prepiriform areas of the cerebral cortex.

A   False
Fractures of the anterior cranial fossa may lead to interruption of the olfactory nerves, and hence bilateral anosmia.

B   False
It is the cribriform plate of the ethmoid bone.

C   False
The olfactory nerves are the central processes of the olfactory cells and not the peripheral processes of a central group of cells. In this respect they differ from other afferent fibres.

D   True
See above.

E   False
Even in the case of bilateral anosmia, the inhalation of vapours from a bottle of concentrated ammonia will stimulate nasal trigeminal sensory receptors and lead to a reaction. Thus the anosmia of a patient who claims to be unaffected by this clinical examination is likely to be spurious. It is recognized that following head injury symptoms may be elaborated pending settlement of compensation claims. Such a compensation or traumatic neurosis may resolve after such a claim is settled.

Question 1.8

The following are midbrain structures:

A substantia nigra

B nucleus ambiguus

C thalamus

D inferior colliculus

E cerebral aqueduct.

Answer 1.8

The midbrain or mesencephalon consists of the following structures:

(i) the tectum, which consists of the corpora quadrigemina, comprised of
- the superior colliculi
- the inferior colliculi

(ii) the basis pedunculi
(iii) the substantia nigra
(iv) the tegmentum, containing
- the red nuclei
- fibre tracts
- grey matter surrounding the cerebral aqueduct

A   True
See above.

B   False
The nucleus ambiguus lies in the medulla oblongata. It is the common motor nucleus of the ninth (glossopharyngeal), tenth (vagus), and eleventh (accessory) cranial nerves.

C   False
The thalamus is a diencephalic structure.

D and E   True
See above.

Question 1.9

Sympathetic stimulation causes:

A release of glucose from the liver
B contraction of the detrusor muscle of the urinary bladder
C increased renal output
D penile erection
E increased blood coagulation.

Answer 1.9

The sympathetic nervous system is that part of the autonomic nervous system that can be thought of as being involved in emergency functions and the response to stress — the 'fight-flight' response. The parasympathetic nervous system, on the other hand, is involved in more 'vegetative' functions, such as the conservation of body resources and the preservation of normal resting functions.

When these general concepts are borne in mind, the effects of sympathetic and parasympathetic stimulation are relatively easy to work out from first principles.

A   True
Important sympathetic effects on hepatic function include the promotion of glycogenolysis, which can be thought of as a way of helping to provide energy in a crisis situation, and the inhibition of bile secretion. The parasympathetic effects, on the other hand, are to stimulate both glycogenesis (thus helping to conserve body resources) and the secretion of bile.

B   False
The contraction of the detrusor muscle of the urinary bladder is a parasympathetic effect. The parasympathetic nervous system also sends inhibitory fibres to the internal sphincter. It would clearly be inappropriate for a strong desire to micturate to be stimulated during the 'fight-flight' response. In fact, the sympathetic nervous system sends inhibitory fibres to the detrusor muscle, and motor fibres to the internal sphincter, the muscle of the upper urethra, and the trigone.

C   False
Sympathetic stimulation causes decreased renal output.

D   False
It is parasympathetic stimulation that leads to penile erection. Sympathetic stimulation causes ejaculation.

E   True
Sympathetic stimulation leads to an increase in the coagulability of the blood, which can be thought of as a preparation for potentional injury during the 'fight-flight' response.

Question 1.10

The following are found in neurones:

A   Golgi apparatus

B   Nissl substance

C   melanin

D   centrioles

E   Barr body.

Answer 1.10

All true
The neuronal nucleus is relatively large and usually possesses one prominent nucleolus. A Barr body occurs in the nuclei of females. The neuronal cytoplasm or neuroplasm is semifluid and viscous and amongst its inclusions are the Nissl substance, Golgi apparatus, mitochondria, microfilaments, microtubules, lysosomes, centrioles, lipofuscin, melanin, glycogen, and lipid.

The Nissl substance is composed of rough endoplasmic reticulum and synthesizes protein. This is transported to the synaptic terminals along the axon via axoplasmic flow. In a process known as chromatolysis the Nissl substance concentrates at the periphery of the cytoplasm following neuronal damage or fatigue and seems to disappear.

The Golgi apparatus is classically demonstrated under the light microscope following staining by osmium or silver impregnation methods. It has the appearance of a reticulum and is probably involved in synthetic activities.

Mitochondria are present throughout the neurone and are involved in energy production. Following section of a spinal nerve there is an increase in the mitochondria of the corresponding anterior horn cells. This reflects an increase in neuronal oxidative phosphorylation.

Microfilaments are arranged in bundles to form the neurofibrils demonstrated by light microscopy.

Microtubules have been shown by electron microscopy to be present throughout the neurone. It has been suggested that they are involved in transport and in the process of axon growth.

Lysosomes are spherical membrane-surrounded bodies containing a number of powerful enzymes. They may act as the neuronal digestive system or as internal scavengers. The inherited lack of a given lysosomal enzyme may lead to the accumulation of material and cause mental disorder. For example, in Niemann–Pick disease there is a deficiency of sphingomyelinase and the accumulation of sphingomyelin. Other so-called storage diseases include Gaucher's disease, Tay–Sach's disease, and glycogen storage disease II.

Lipofuscin is a lysosomal metabolic product which accumulates with age and with nervous system trauma or disease. It is thought to be harmless.

Melanin is a brown to black pigment found in the cytoplasm of neurones in, for example, the substantia nigra and the locus coeruleus.

Question 1.11

Constriction of the pupil with accommodation requires the following structures to be intact:

A   optic nerve
B   optic tract
C   cerebral cortex
D   lateral geniculate nucleus
E   stellate ganglion.

Answer 1.11

The eye focuses on near objects through the process of accommodation, whereby the circular and longitudinal fibres of the ciliary muscle contract and so allow the lens of the eye to become more spherical passively. This process is accompanied by reflex ocular convergence, through contraction of the medial recti muscles, in order to allow the retinal images to continue to be focused on the same parts of each retina. In addition, there is reflex pupillary constriction, which helps diminish the light falling on the peripheral part of the lens, in order to reduce the optical aberrations that are more likely to occur as the lens adopts a more spherical shape. The convergence originates in the cortex and is relayed to the ciliary muscles via the oculomotor nuclei.

A   False
The optic nerve is not involved in this pupillary reflex. However, it *is* involved in the direct pupillary light reflex.

B   False
The optic tract is not involved in this pupillary reflex. As in the case of the optic nerve, it is involved in the direct pupillary light reflex.

C   True
See above.

D   False
The lateral geniculate nucleus is not involved in the constriction of the pupil with accommodation. As in the case of the optic nerve and tract, however, it is involved in the direct pupillary light reflex.

E   False
The stellate ganglion is formed by the first thoracic ganglion joining the inferior cervical ganglion and is not involved in this pupillary reflex.

Question 1.12

The corticospinal tracts:

A   are also known as the pyramidal tracts

B   decussate in the midbrain

C   run in the posterior limb of the internal capsule

D   originate mainly from the postcentral cortex

E   degenerate in tabes dorsalis.

Answer 1.12

The corticospinal tracts provide the upper motor neurones. Their fibres originate from the pyramidal cells of the motor cortex and transmit voluntary motor information to the lower motor neurones that pass from the spinal cord to muscles, via the anterior spinal roots. The anterior corticospinal tracts, also known as the direct pyramidal or uncrossed motor tracts, are small tracts that are confined to the cervical and superior thoracic region of the spinal cord. The lateral corticospinal tracts are also known as the pyramidal or crossed motor tracts and, unlike the anterior corticospinal tracts, they decussate in the medulla oblongata and then pass inferiorly on the contralateral side of the spinal cord. At each spinal segment fibres leave the lateral corticospinal tracts to enter the anterior grey columns of the spinal cord and synapse with lower motor neurones. Thus the tracts diminish in size inferiorly.

A True
See above.

B False
See above.

C True
The fibres run from the cerebral cortex to the internal capsule via the corona radiata. They occupy the anterior two-thirds of the posterior limb of the internal capsule, and the posterior third of the anterior limb.

D False
They originate mainly from the precentral motor area of the cerebral cortex.

E False
In tabes dorsalis, also known as locomotor ataxia, syphilitic infection leads to degeneration of the central processes of dorsal root ganglion cells and of the posterior or dorsal white columns of the spinal cord.

Question 1.13

The spinothalamic tracts convey sensory impulses concerned with:

A discriminative touch

B pain

C conscious proprioception

D temperature

E vibration.

Answer 1.13

A   False
The anterior or ventral spinothalamic tracts convey crude touch sensations. Discriminative touch, however, is conveyed by the ipsilateral posterior or dorsal white columns, known as the gracile and cuneate fasciculi.

B   True
Pain sensations are conveyed by the contralateral lateral spinothalamic tracts.

C   False
It is true that some fibres originating from joint receptors reach the dorsal horn and after synapse the impulses are carried across the spinal cord to the contralateral spinothalamic tracts. However, it is the ipsilateral posterior white columns that are responsible for conveying conscious muscle sense concerned with the appreciation of body position.

D   True
Temperature sensations are carried by the contralateral lateral spinothalamic tracts.

E   False
Vibration sense is conveyed by the ipsilateral posterior white columns.

Question 1.14

The following statements concerning the spinal cord are true:

A the posterior spinal artery supplies the posterior three-quarters of the spinal cord

B in the adult it has an average length of approximately 30 cm

C prior to adolescence the spinal cord is relatively shorter in comparison with the vertebral column than in the adult

D in the adult it terminates at the level of the inferior border of the third lumbar vertebra

E there are 30 pairs of spinal nerves.

Answer 1.14

All false

The spinal cord is contained within the vertebral column and is continuous superiorly with the medulla oblongata of the brainstem through the foramen magnum of the skull. In the adult it is on average approximately 45 cm long, terminating inferiorly at the level of the inferior border of the first lumbar vertebra. Prior to adolescence the spinal cord is relatively longer in comparison with the vertebral column, reaching the level of the third lumbar vertebra at birth, and being the length of the entire vertebral canal at three months after conception.

Thirty-one pairs of spinal nerves are attached to the spinal cord via the anterior or ventral motor roots and the posterior or dorsal sensory roots. The cell bodies of the sensory neurones are in the posterior (or dorsal) root ganglia. The cell bodies of the lower motor neurones which give rise to the anterior motor roots are in the anterior grey columns of the spinal cord itself. The internal organisation of the spinal cord demonstrates an inner H-shaped core of grey matter surrounded by white matter. The grey matter is divided into anterior, lateral, and posterior columns or horns, and a central connecting grey commissure. The white matter is mainly made up of myelinated fibres, and is similarly divided into anterior, lateral, and posterior columns.

The spinal cord is divided into five regions on the basis of the site of exit from the vertebral column of the 31 pairs of spinal nerves. Starting superiorly these are: cervical (eight pairs), thoracic (twelve pairs), lumbar (five pairs), sacral (five pairs), and coccygeal (one pair).

The anterior spinal artery supplies the anterior two-thirds of the spinal cord and the posterior spinal artery supplies the posterior one-third.

The two most important functions of the spinal cord are, firstly, the transmission of impulses to and from the brain via the ascending and descending tracts, and secondly, the mediation of spinal cord reflexes.

Question 1.15

Dendrites:

A do not contain Nissl substance

B are usually covered with myelin

C usually number more than one per neurone

D provide an important part of the neuronal receptor surface

E provide the site of origin of some axons.

Answer 1.15

The cell body or soma of the neurone is known as the perikaryon or neurocyte. Projecting from the perikaryon are two types of neurite, the axon and the dendrite. The dendrites are responsible for receiving information and carrying it to the perikaryon.

A False
The Nissl substance, which is involved in protein synthesis, is present in dendrites but absent in the axon.

B False
It is the axon which may be ensheathed in the lamellated interrupted covering known as the myelin sheath. These interruptions are the nodes of Ranvier, and the segments between the nodes are known as internodes. The proximal axon segment, the axon hillock, is unmyelinated and is, in many neurones, the site of initiation of the action potential. Myelination ceases at the distal end of the axon, which may be branched with terminal boutons.

C True
Dendrites differ from axons in that there is usually more than one per neurone.

D True
Dendrites are usually branched and studded with dendritic spines, which are sites of synaptic contact.

E True
There is usually one axon per neurone, and it takes origin from the perikaryon or from one of the main dendrites.

Question 1.16

Cell bodies within the nuclei of origin of the following cranial nerves give rise to preganglionic parasympathetic fibres:

A oculomotor

B trigeminal

C glossopharyngeal

D facial

E hypoglossal.

Answer 1.16

A True
The accessory parasympathetic or Edinger–Westphal nucleus of the oculomotor (III) cranial nerve lies posterior to the main nucleus. Its preganglionic parasympathetic fibres pass to the ciliary ganglion where they synapse. The postganglionic parasympathetic fibres pass to the ciliary muscles and constrictor pupillae via the short ciliary nerves.

B False
The trigeminal nerve (V) is the largest cranial nerve and has the following four nuclei:
  (i) the main sensory nucleus, which is in the posterior pons;
 (ii) the spinal nucleus, which is continuous with the above nucleus superiorly, and passes through the medulla inferiorly to C2;
(iii) the mesencephalic nucleus, which is in the grey matter surrounding the cerebral aqueduct, and passes inferiorly into the pons;
 (iv) the motor nucleus, which is in the pons.

C True
The parasympathetic or inferior salivary nucleus of the glossopharyngeal nerve (IX) lies inferior to the superior salivary nucleus, and close to the superior tip of the nucleus ambiguus. It receives inputs from the hypothalamus, olfactory system, tractus solitarius nucleus, and trigeminal sensory nucleus. Preganglionic fibres from this nucleus enter the tympanic branch of the glossopharyngeal nerve and reach the otic ganglion via the tympanic plexus and the lesser petrosal nerve. Postganglionic fibres supply the parotid gland via the auriculotemporal branch of the mandibular nerve.

D True
The parasympathetic or lacrimal and superior salivary nuclei of the facial nerve (VII) lie posterolateral to the main motor nucleus of this cranial nerve. The lacrimal nucleus supplies the lacrimal gland. The superior salivary nucleus supplies the nasal and palatine glands, and the sublingual and submandibular salivary glands.

E False
There is no parasympathetic component to the nucleus of the hypoglossal nerve (XII) which is in the floor of the fourth ventricle and supplies all the extrinsic and intrinsic muscles of the tongue, with the exception of the palatoglossus muscle.

FURTHER READING

Emslie-Smith D, Paterson C R, Scratcherd T, Read N W (editors) 1988
Textbook of physiology, 11th edn. Churchill Livingstone, Edinburgh
Kaplan H I, Sadock B J (editors) 1989 Comprehensive textbook of
psychiatry, 5th edn. Williams and Wilkins, Baltimore (Chapter on
Neural Science)
Kendell R E, Zealley A K (editors) 1988 Companion to psychiatric studies,
4th edn. Churchill Livingstone, Edinburgh (Chapter on Functional
Neuroanatomy)
Rubenstein D, Wayne D 1985 Lecture notes on clinical medicine, 3rd
edn. Blackwell Scientific, Oxford (Part 1: The Clinical Approach —
Chapter on the Nervous System)
Snell R S 1987 Clinical neuroanatomy for medical students, 2nd edn.
Little, Brown and Company, Boston
Walton J 1985 Brain's diseases of the nervous system, 9th edn. Oxford
University Press, Oxford
Williams P L, Warwick R, Dyson M, Bannister L H (editors) 1989 Gray's
anatomy, 37th edn. Churchill Livingstone, Edinburgh (Section on
Neurology, pp 859–1244)

2. Neuropathology and neurology

Syllabus requirements

In neuropathology the candidate's knowledge of the principal neuropathological changes in degenerative disorders, cerebrovascular disorders, and other conditions which may be referred to the psychiatrist should be updated as the basis of neurological examination and diagnosis.

Question 2.1

Papilloedema is a feature of:

A meningitis
B benign intracranial hypertension
C Wilson's disease
D malignant hypertension
E optic neuritis.

Answer 2.1

Papilloedema is swelling of the optic nerve head (optic disc). The disc is pinker than usual in the early stages, with the veins appearing full. This is followed by blurring of the nasal margin of the optic disc which spreads to the temporal margin. At the same time the physiological cup fills with exudate and thus becomes obliterated. The surface of the optic disc may become raised owing to the swelling. Severe papilloedema of acute onset may be accompanied by areas of haemorrhage. The optic disc may become paler in chronic papilloedema as a result of optic atrophy.

A   True
Meningitis can cause papilloedema through the mechanism of raised intracranial pressure. The latter leads to a rise in cerebrospinal fluid pressure which enlarges the subarachnoid space around the optic nerve, and so causes retinal venous compression. Other intracranial lesions that can also lead to papilloedema by the same means include intracranial tumours and cerebral abscesses.

B   True
Benign intracranial hypertension can produce papilloedema by the mechanism described in **A** above.

C   False
A pathognomonic ophthalmic sign of Wilson's disease is the Kayser–Fleischer ring. This is a zone of golden-brown, yellow or green corneal pigmentation caused by the deposition of copper.

D   True
In papilloedema secondary to malignant hypertension there is blurring of the margin of the optic disc and sometimes exudate in the physiological cup, as described above. However, it is rare for the optic disc to be very swollen. In addition, arterial thickening and areas of white exudate may be seen in the retina.

E   True
When papilloedema is caused by inflammatory lesions of the optic nerve such as optic neuritis, it may then be referred to as papillitis.

Question 2.2

Cerebellar lesions may cause:

A a static tremor

B nystagmus which is less marked when looking towards the side of the lesion

C Rombergism

D dysarthria

E muscular hypertonicity.

Answer 2.2

A destructive cerebellar lesion gives rise to ipsilateral signs.
These signs may be almost as severe following destruction of
the superior cerebellar peduncle or dentate nucleus as following
damage to a whole cerebellar hemisphere.

A   True
A static tremor may occur when the patient attempts to maintain
a limb in a fixed position. Cerebellar lesions also give rise to an
intention tremor, which can be demonstrated by the finger–nose
test.

B   False
Nystagmus is usually present and is more marked when looking
towards the side of the lesion.

C   False
Rombergism or a positive Romberg's sign is present if a patient,
on being asked to stand with his or her feet together, is more
unsteady with closed eyes than with the eyes open. It is caused
by loss of postural sensibility in the lower limbs which can be
compensated for by vision. It is seen in tabes dorsalis. Standing
may be difficult or impossible following a cerebellar lesion,
especially one affecting the midline vermis. The cause in this
case is truncal ataxia and Rombergism is not present.

D   True
The patient may appear to be drunk, with speech that is jerky
and explosive with individual syllables being slurred.

E   False
In cerebellar lesions there is muscular hypotonia owing to loss
of the cerebellar influence on the stretch reflex.

Question 2.3

Recognised features of Bell's palsy include:

A hyperacusis

B anosmia

C change in sense of taste

D the crocodile tears phenomenon

E a pleocytosis in the cerebrospinal fluid.

Answer 2.3

Bell's palsy is a paralysis of the facial or seventh cranial nerve and is named after Sir Charles Bell (1774–1842). The facial paralysis is usually unilateral and of sudden onset.

A   True
If the facial nerve lesion is proximal to the nerve to the stapedius muscle then the patient may suffer from an unpleasant intensification of loud sounds.

B   False
This can occur with lesions to the olfactory or first cranial nerves.

C   True
Loss of the sense of taste on the anterior two-thirds of the tongue can occur when the facial nerve lesion is proximal to the chorda tympani. In such cases a decrease in salivation also occurs.

D   True
The crocodile tears phenomenon can occur during recovery if regenerating autonomic fibres wrongly innervate the lacrimal glands rather than the salivary glands that were originally innervated by them.

E   False
This can occur in poliomyelitis. Its importance lies in the fact that this disease may closely simulate Bell's palsy and may therefore have to be considered in the differential diagnosis, especially when the sudden unilateral facial paralysis occurs during a poliomyelitis epidemic. Another condition that may also present in a similar way is multiple sclerosis.

Question 2.4

A reduction in the cerebrospinal fluid glucose concentration characteristically occurs in the following:

A fungal meningitis

B bacterial meningitis

C viral meningitis

D carcinomatous meningitis

E diabetes mellitus.

Answer 2.4

The normal concentration of glucose in the cerebrospinal fluid is between 2.2 and 4.5 mM (40–80 mg/100 ml).

A True
Fungal meningitis characteristically causes a marked reduction in the glucose concentration.

B True
As in the above case, a marked reduction of glucose concentration is also a characteristic of bacterial meningitis.

C False
The glucose concentration is usually normal in viral meningitis.

D True
Carcinomatous meningitis causes a moderate reduction in the glucose concentration.

E False
The cerebrospinal fluid glucose concentration is approximately 1.7 mM less than the blood glucose concentration. Thus a high glucose level in the cerebrospinal fluid may be found in diabetes mellitus.

Question 2.5

Meningiomas are commonly:

A malignant

B derived from cortical cells

C found below the tentorium

D found along the course of the intracranial venous sinuses

E associated with hyperostosis.

Answer 2.5

Meningiomas are extracerebral tumours which are almost always benign, encapsulated, and attached to the dura mater. They are usually removable surgically.

A   False
See above.

B   False
Meningiomas are thought to be derived from the arachnoid cells of the arachnoid villi.

C   False
Meningiomas are rarely found below the tentorium.

D   True
Because they arise from arachnoid villus cells meningiomas are commonly found along the course of the intracranial venous sinuses. Their commonest sites of origin are:

- the sphenoidal ridges
- the convexities of the hemispheres
- the suprasellar region
- the olfactory groove.

E   True
Meningiomas are usually closely related to the skull and hyperostosis results from invasion of the overlying bony tissue by the tumour.

Question 2.6

Features of dysfunction of the frontal lobe include:

A cortical sensory loss

B alexia

C polydipsia

D dyscalculia

E increased initiative.

Answer 2.6

Features of the frontal lobe syndrome include the following:

- Change of personality, with, for example
  — disinhibition
  — reduced social and ethical control
  — sexual indiscretions
  — financial and personal errors of judgement
  — elevated mood
  — irritability
- Impaired attention, concentration, and initiative
- Aspontaneity, and slowed psychomotor activity
- Orbital lesions may cause
  — anosmia
  — ipsilateral optic atrophy
- When the motor cortex is affected there may be
  — contralateral spastic paresis
  — grasp reflex
  — increased tendon reflexes
  — positive Babinski sign
  — gait decompensation
- Posterior dominant frontal lobe lesions may cause
  — apraxia of the face and tongue
  — primary motor aphasia
  — motor agraphia
- Motor Jacksonian fits
- Incontinence, usually urinary.

A   False
Cortical sensory loss is a feature of parietal lobe dysfunction.

B   False
Alexia is a feature of dominant temporal lobe dysfunction.

C   False
Polydipsia is a feature of hypothalamic dysfunction.

D   False
Dyscalculia is a feature of dominant parietal lobe dysfunction.

E   False
Impaired initiative is seen in frontal lobe dysfunction (see above).

Question 2.7

Features of dysfunction of the parietal lobe include:

A contralateral homonymous hemianopia

B dressing apraxia

C finger agnosia

D hypersomnia

E constructional apraxia.

Answer 2.7

Features of parietal lobe dysfunction include:

- Visuospatial difficulties such as constructional apraxia and visuospatial agnosia
- Topographical disorientation
- Cortical sensory loss
- Visual inattention
- Sensory Jacksonian fits
- Dominant parietal lobe lesions may cause
  — Gerstmann's syndrome
  — primary motor aphasia (anterior lesions)
  — primary sensory aphasia (posterior lesions) including agraphia and alexia
  — motor apraxia
  — bilateral tactile agnosia
  — visual agnosia (parieto-occipital lesions)
- Non-dominant parietal lobe lesions may cause
  — anosognosia
  — dressing apraxia
  — hemisomatognosia
  — prosopagnosia

A   False
Contralateral homonymous hemianopia is seen in temporal lobe dysfunction.

B   True
See above.

C   True
Finger agnosia is part of Gerstmann's syndrome, other features of which include dyscalculia, agraphia, and right-left disorientation.

D   False
Causes of hypersomnia include narcolepsy, sleep apnoea, the Pickwickian syndrome, and the Kleine–Levin syndrome.
Hypersomnia is sometimes defined as a tendency to sleep which can be resisted; narcolepsy, in which there are day-time attacks of irresistable sleep, would not therefore be included under this definition.

E   True
See above.

Question 2.8

Features of dysfunction of the temporal lobe include:

A schizophrenia-like psychosis

B amnesia

C emotional lability

D contralateral spastic paresis

E lower quadrant contralateral homonymous hemianopia.

Answer 2.8

Features of dysfunction of the temporal lobe include the following:

- Dominant temporal lobe lesions may cause
  — sensory aphasia
  — alexia
  — agraphia
- Posterior dominant temporal lobe lesions may cause features of the parietal lobe syndrome
- Non-dominant temporal lobe lesions may cause
  — hemisomatognosia
  — prosopagnosia
  — visuospatial difficulties
  — impaired retention and learning of non-verbal patterned stimuli such as music
- Bilateral medial temporal lobe lesions may cause amnesic syndromes
- Personality changes may occur which are similar to those caused by frontal lobe lesions
- Psychosis
- Epilepsy
- Contralateral homonymous upper quadrantic visual field defect.

A   True
Flor-Henry (1969) reported an association between schizophrenia and dominant temporal lobe epilepsy, and between mood (or affective) disorder and non-dominant temporal lobe epilepsy.

B   True
See above.

C   True
See above.

D   False
Contralateral spastic paresis may result from dysfunction of the motor cortex.

E   False
The visual field defect is an upper quadrant contralateral homonymous hemianopia.

Question 2.9

Neurofibrillary tangles in the cerebral cortex

A can be demonstrated by silver staining

B consist of abnormal neurites surrounding an amyloid core

C are often widespread in Down's syndrome

D are often widespread in normal old age

E correlate in number with the degree of cognitive impairment.

Answer 2.9

Neurofibrillary tangles are widespread in the cerebral cortex in senile dementia of the Alzheimer type. They can be demonstrated under the light microscope in frozen or paraffin sections stained by silver impregnation techniques. They have been found to consist of twisted helically paired filaments, and there is evidence that their number correlates with the degree of cognitive impairment.

A True
See above.

B False
It is neuritic plaques that consist of abnormal neurites surrounding an amyloid core. Like neurofibrillary tangles, neuritic plaques (formerly known as senile plaques) are also a characteristic neuropathological feature of senile dementia of the Alzheimer type.

C True
The neuropathological features of patients with Down's syndrome who survive into adulthood bear a marked similarity to those found in senile dementia of the Alzheimer type. This has led to speculation over the years on the possibility of common pathology or some element of shared aetiology between the two conditions, and indeed recent advances in molecular genetics indicate that genetic information of importance to the pathogenesis Alzheimer's disease lies on chromosome 21. Other conditions in which neurofibrillary tangles are common include post-encephalitic parkinsonism and the parkinsonism-dementia complex of Guam.

D False
Neurofibrillary tangles are seen only occasionally in the cerebral cortex in normal old age.

E True
See above.

Question 2.10

Characteristic features of the Argyll–Robertson pupil in neurosyphilis include:

A   intact ciliospinal reflex

B   contraction on convergence

C   contraction to light

D   wide dilatation

E   depigmentation of the iris.

Answer 2.10

Argyll–Robertson pupils in neurosyphilis are small, irregular and unequal in size, and do not react to light. The iris is typically atrophied and depigmented. When the cause is congenital syphilis, Argyll–Robertson pupils may be dilated.

A   False
In the intact ciliospinal reflex when the skin on one side of the neck is scratched there is dilatation of the ipsilateral pupil. This reflex is lost in Argyll–Robertson pupils caused by neurosyphilis.

B   True
The convergence reflex of the normal eye is retained.

C and D   False
See above.

E   True
See above.

Question 2.11

Characteristic neuropathological features of Pick's disease include:

A neuronal loss most marked in the inner layers of the cortex

B astrocytic proliferation

C knife blade atrophy of the gyri

D selective parietal lobe atrophy

E ballooned cells.

Answer 2.11

A False
The neuronal loss in Pick's disease is most marked in the outer layers of the cortex.

B True
Cortical and subcortical astrocytic proliferation and fibrous gliosis are seen on histological examination.

C True
Knife blade atrophy of the gyri is seen in this disease.

D False
There is asymmetrical selective atrophy of the temporal lobes and the adjacent inferior and medial surfaces of the frontal lobes. It is unusual for there to be major involvement of the parietal lobes.

E True
Ballooned cells are a characteristic histopathological feature of Pick's disease and consist of swollen oval neurones which have lost their Nissl substance and which have silver staining inclusions known as Pick bodies.

Question 2.12

Characteristic features of multi-infarct dementia include:

A insidious onset
B focal neurological symptoms and signs
C ventricular dilatation
D history of hypertension
E gradual deterioration.

Answer 2.12

Multi-infarct dementia, also known as arteriosclerotic dementia, shows the following pathological features:

- arteriosclerosis of major arteries
- local or general atrophy
- cerebral infarction
- ventricular dilatation
- multiple infarcted areas related in extent to the degree of cognitive impairment
- multiple ischaemic areas
- gliosis

Multi-infarct dementia is commoner in men. There is usually a history of hypertension with related clinical features. The onset is typically acute, and the deterioration stepwise. Focal neurological symptoms and signs occur, and there may be nocturnal confusion and fluctuating cognitive impairment. Emotional incontinence and low mood are also seen.

Thus the correct answers are:

A   False

B   True

C   True

D   True

E   False.

Question 2.13

Characteristic features of Creutzfeldt–Jakob disease include:

A   gross atrophy of the cerebral cortex

B   degeneration of spinal cord long descending tracts

C   status spongiosus

D   myoclonic jerks

E   neuritic plaques.

Answer 2.13

A False
There is usually little or no gross atrophy of the cerebral cortex
in Creutzfeldt–Jakob disease, although in patients who survive
longer than a year there is sometimes diffuse cerebral atrophy.
Most patients, however, die within 3 months and 1 year of the
onset. In cases of longer survival there may also be evidence of
selective cerebellar atrophy. Ventricular dilatation is common.

B True
The corticospinal tracts and extrapyramidal pathways are often
severely degenerated.

C True
Status spongiosus of the grey matter of the cortex is highly
characteristic of Creutzfeldt–Jakob disease. It is so-called because
on histological examination tissue that is affected has a spongy
appearance. It should be noted that status spongiosus is not
pathognomonic for Creutzfeldt–Jakob disease; this histological
change has been reported in certain other degenerative
conditions such as senile dementia of the Alzheimer type, Pick's
disease, and Wilson's disease.

D True
There is a progressive dementia which is frequently
accompanied by myoclonic jerks. Other clinical features vary a
great deal from case to case.

E False
Neuritic plaques are rare in Creutzfeldt–Jakob disease. They are
a characteristic neuropathological feature of senile dementia of
the Alzheimer type.

Question 2.14

Characteristic features of the punch-drunk syndrome include:

A dilated ventricles

B neurofibrillary tangles

C dysarthria

D pyramidal lesions

E personality deterioration.

Answer 2.14

The punch-drunk syndrome, or chronic traumatic encephalopathy, may occur in those who are subjected to repeated blows to the head, for example professional boxers. Neuropathological features include cerebral atrophy and sometimes perforation of the septum pellucidum.

Clinical features include:

- cerebellar features
- extrapyramidal features
- pyramidal features
- impairment of memory and intellect
- deterioration of personality.

A True

There is characteristically enlargement of the lateral ventricles.

B True

Neurofibrillary tangles, similar to those seen in senile dementia of the Alzheimer type, are typically widespread throughout the cerebral cortex and brain stem. However, the neuritic plaques of Alzheimer's disease are rare.

C True

Dysarthria is one of the principal features of the condition, including mild cases.

D True

Evidence of asymmetrical pyramidal lesions is commonly present from an early stage.

E True

See above.

Question 2.15

Characteristic features of normal pressure hydrocephalus include:

A headache

B disturbance of gait

C ventricular enlargement secondary to cerebral atrophy

D onset in infancy

E progressive dementia.

Answer 2.15

Hydrocephalus, a diffuse enlargement of the ventricular system, can be divided into:

- obstructive
  - a block exists to the circulation of the cerebrospinal fluid
  - usually non-communicating: that is, the ventricles do not communicate freely with the subarachnoid space
- non-obstructive
  - the ventricular enlargement is secondary to cerebral atrophy
  - communicating

In normal pressure hydrocephalus the situation is different to the above types with the hydrocephalus being both obstructive and communicating. Other names include occult hydrocephalus, communicating hydrocephalus, and hydrocephalic dementia. Normal pressure hydrocephalus is caused by a block in the subarachnoid space which prevents the cerebrospinal fluid from being reabsorbed.

A   False
The pressure in the ventricular system is often normal, so that features such as headache are usually absent.

B   True
Other features that typically occur in normal pressure hydrocephalus include progressive dementia and urinary incontinence or urgency. Whilst the latter may only occur later in the course of this condition, the disturbance of gait may actually be the presenting feature.

C   False
Ventricular enlargement is secondary to cerebral atrophy in non-obstructive hydrocephalus. There have been a number of theories to explain how ventricular enlargement occurs in normal pressure hydrocephalus when the pressure in the ventricular system is often normal in this condition. For further information see the textbook by Lishman (1987).

D   False
Normal pressure hydrocephalus predominantly affects patients in their 60s and 70s.

E   True
See the answer to **B** above.

Question 2.16

Infarctions in the distribution of the anterior cerebral artery lead to:

A motor aphasia

B contralateral hemianopia

C ipsilateral Horner's syndrome

D contralateral hemiplegia

E body image disturbances.

Answer 2.16

Infarctions in the distribution of the anterior cerebral artery lead to:

- contralateral hemiparesis (leg affected more severely than the arm)
- grasp reflex
- motor aphasia
- cortical sensory loss
- clouding of consciousness
- personality change of the frontal lobe dysfunction type
- changes in mental functioning similar to those seen in a global dementia
- incontinence.

A   True
See above.

B   False
Contralateral hemianopia is an effect of posterior cerebral artery infarction.

C   False
An ipsilateral Horner's syndrome can result from occlusion of the internal carotid artery, as a result of involvement of the carotid sheath sympathetic fibres.

D   True
See above.

E   False
Agnosic syndromes and body image disturbances can result from lesions to the non-dominant cerebral hemisphere following occlusion of the corresponding middle cerebral artery.

FURTHER READING

Adams J H, Graham D I 1988 An introduction to neuropathology. Churchill Livingstone, Edinburgh

Bannister R 1985 Brain's clinical neurology, 6th edn. Oxford University Press, Oxford

Flor-Henry P 1969 Psychosis and temporal lobe epilepsy: a controlled investigation. Epilepsia 10: 363–395

Kaplan H I, Sadock B J (editors) 1989 Comprehensive textbook of psychiatry, 5th edn. Williams and Wilkins, Baltimore (Chapters on Neural Science and Neurology)

Lindsay K W, Bone I, Callander R 1986 Neurology and neurosurgery illustrated. Churchill Livingstone, Edinburgh

Lishman W A 1987 Organic psychiatry: the psychological consequences of cerebral disorder, 2nd edn. Blackwell Scientific, Oxford

Rubenstein D, Wayne D 1985 Lecture notes on clinical medicine, 3rd edn. Blackwell Scientific, Oxford (Part 1: The clinical approach — chapter on the Nervous System; and Part 2: Essential background information — chapter on Neurology)

Walton J 1985 Brain's diseases of the nervous system, 9th edn. Oxford University Press, Oxford

Williams P L, Warwick R, Dyson M, Bannister L H (editors) 1989 Gray's anatomy, 37th edn. Churchill Livingstone, Edinburgh (Section on neurology, pp 859–1244)

3. Clinical psychopharmacology

Syllabus requirements

Basic principles of pharmacokinetics and drug action and interaction should be revised in relation to the main groups of drugs used in psychiatry — anxiolytics, antidepressives, antipsychotics, sedatives/hypnotics, lithium and anticonvulsants. What is required is an understanding of the pharmacological principles relevant to the prescribing of drugs in psychiatry.

(The methodology of clinical trials is part of the MRCPsych Part II syllabus.)

Question 3.1

Following oral administration drugs are characteristically absorbed:

A mainly in the stomach unless they are enteric coated

B primarily by active transport

C better when in the ionised form

D less readily in the presence of food in the gut

E more slowly than when given by intramuscular injection.

Answer 3.1

The major mechanisms for absorption of drugs from the alimentary tract are:

- passive diffusion
- pore filtration
- active transport

Most drugs are absorbed by passive diffusion through the bimolecular lipid sheet. Most are too large to pass across by pore filtration, and most do not fulfil the appropriate specific structural criteria to be carried by active transport systems.

Factors which influence absorption include:

- gastric emptying
- gastric pH
- intestinal motility
- food in the alimentary canal
- intestinal microflora
- area of absorption
- blood flow.

A   False
The small intestine is the primary site of absorption of orally administered drugs. Gastric absorption of any importance only occurs with ethanol and weak acids. Enteric coating is used either to protect a drug from gastric acid or to protect the stomach from harmful drug side-effects.

B   False
See above.

C   False
Transfer by passive diffusion across the bimolecular lipid sheet occurs more readily when a drug is in the unionised form.

D   False
The presence of food can lead to increased absorption for many drugs, such as diazepam, metoprolol, propranolol, hydralazine, and hydrochlorothiazide.

E   True
Intramuscular injection results in a more rapid onset of action than the oral route.

Question 3.2

With regard to the transfer of substances from the blood to the cerebrospinal fluid:

A it occurs primarily by passive diffusion in the case of purines

B it occurs primarily by passive diffusion in the case of levodopa

C it increases as the pK_a of a drug becomes very low

D there is little or no transfer of adrenaline and amphetamine

E it is better the more water-soluble a drug is.

Answer 3.2

The transfer of substances from the blood to the cerebrospinal fluid is limited by the blood–brain barrier. Some astrocytic processes end as perivascular feet on capillaries and it is this gliovascular membrane that helps to form the barrier.

In general there is a high rate of penetration of the blood–brain barrier for nonpolar highly lipid-soluble drugs. The penetration of highly polar water-soluble drugs is low or non-existent.

A False
Active transport mechanisms are involved in the transfer across the blood–brain barrier of essential nutrients such as purines, pyrimidines, amino acids, and glucose.

B False
As an amino acid precursor of dopamine, levodopa is treated as an essential nutrient and crosses the blood–brain barrier by active transport. On the other hand, dopamine is unable to cross the blood–brain barrier under normal circumstances. Hence the rationale for using levodopa in the treatment of the functional deficiency of dopamine in Parkinson's disease.

C False
The stronger an acidic (lower pK_a) or basic (higher pK_a) drug, the slower is the rate of penetration of the blood–brain barrier, because of the higher degree of ionisation.

D False
The statement is true for the more polar, and therefore less lipid-soluble, adrenaline. However, amphetamine, which lacks -OH groups, is less polar than adrenaline, and so is better able to cross the blood–brain barrier. Hence the neuropsychiatric effects of amphetamine.

E False
See above.

Question 3.3

For a drug whose elimination is first order:

A the half-life increases as the dose administered increases

B the rate of elimination is constant

C linear kinetics are obeyed

D the steady state plasma level is proportional to the dose

E the half-life is proportional to the plasma concentration.

Answer 3.3

In first-order elimination the rate of elimination of a drug is directly proportional to the plasma concentration of the drug at a given time. This is also known as linear kinetics, and can be represented mathematically as

$$dC/dt = -kC$$

where C is the plasma concentration of the drug, k is a constant, and t represents time.

The elimination half-life, $t_\frac{1}{2}$, is the time taken for a given value of C to fall to $\frac{1}{2}C$. It can be shown that

$$t_\frac{1}{2} = \ln 2/k$$

where $\ln 2$ is the natural logarithm of 2 and has a fixed value (0.6931 to 4 significant figures).

Thus it follows that the elimination half-life is constant in first-order elimination.

A   False
The elimination half-life is constant.

B   False
As noted above, the rate of elimination of the drug is directly proportional to its plasma concentration. It is in zero-order elimination, also known as saturation kinetics, that the rate of elimination is constant.

C   True
See above.

D   True
It can be shown mathematically that one of the consequences of first-order elimination kinetics is that the steady state plasma level is proportional to the dose.

E   False
See above.

Question 3.4

The volume of distribution of a drug:

A has a specific physiological meaning

B can exceed the total body volume

C is directly proportional to the plasma concentration

D can be stated in units of kilograms per litre

E tends to be higher in drugs that are highly protein bound.

Answer 3.4

The volume of distribution of a drug is conventionally represented by the symbol V_d and is a proportionality constant that relates dose to plasma concentration:

$$V_d = D/C$$

where D is the mass of drug in the body at a given time and C is the corresponding plasma concentration of the drug.

The volume of distribution is a conceptual compartment, having neither an anatomical nor a physiological meaning. It is only very rarely that the volume of distribution may actually correspond to an anatomical space.

A   False
See above.

B   True
The volume of distribution of a drug can exceed the total body volume if there is a heavy concentration of the drug in a particular type of tissue. In adults the volume of distribution may have a value of well over 300 litres for certain drugs.

C   False
It can be seen from the formula above that the volume of distribution is inversely proportional to the plasma concentration.

D   False
Strictly speaking, the volume of distribution has units of volume. However, because its value can vary with body mass, the volume of distribution of a drug is often given in units of volume per kilogram body mass.

E   False
In general, the volume of distribution tends to be lower in drugs that are highly protein bound, and higher in drugs that have a higher lipid solubility. In the latter case such drugs are clearly better able to enter adipose tissue, for example.

Question 3.5

The following statements are true concerning diazepam:

A its plasma protein binding is low

B intramuscular absorption is better than oral absorption

C temazepam is a metabolite

D the liver is the main site of metabolism

E it causes significant hepatic enzyme induction.

Answer 3.5

A   False
The plasma protein binding of diazepam is high, being approximately 95%.

B   False
Benzodiazepines are normally absorbed well when administered orally. However, intramuscular administration is less rapid than oral administration and usually leads to lower peak plasma concentrations.

C   True
Another important metabolite of diazepam is desmethyldiazepam (also known as nordiazepam) which in turn is metabolised to oxazepam.

D   True
Hepatic oxidation is involved in the metabolism of long acting benzodiazepines such as diazepam whilst non-oxidative pathways are important for shorter acting benzodiazepines.

E   False
The benzodiazepines do not significantly induce hepatic microsomal enzymes.

Question 3.6

Imipramine has the following pharmacokinetic properties:
A it is highly lipid soluble
B plasma protein binding is low
C it has a long half-life
D its main metabolite is nortriptyline
E it undergoes a low level of first pass metabolism when taken orally.

Answer 3.6

A True
The tricyclic antidepressants are in general lipid soluble and therefore readily absorbed from the gastrointestinal tract. This is related to the large volume of distribution that the tricyclic antidepressants have; for imipramine values have been found to be in the range 28–61 l/kg body mass.

B False
In general the plasma protein binding of the tricyclic antidepressants is high. The figure for imipramine is approximately 85%. The high protein binding and large volume of distribution leads to poor dialysability following overdosage.

C True
The long half-life makes feasible once daily administration.

D False
The main metabolite of imipramine is desipramine, which is active. Nortriptyline is an active metabolite of amitriptyline. Both these antidepressant metabolites are monomethyl derivatives that result from demethylation of the side-chain of the parent tricyclic antidepressants.

E False
Orally administered imipramine undergoes extensive first pass hepatic metabolism of over 50%.

Question 3.7

Recognised side-effects of phenytoin include:

A thrombocytopenia

B aplastic anaemia

C hyperventilation

D acne

E gingival tenderness.

Answer 3.7

A True
Recognised haematological side-effects of phenytoin include:

- agranulocytosis
- aplastic anaemia
- leucopenia
- megaloblastic anaemia
- thrombocytopenia.

B True
See answer to **A** above.

C False
This is not a recognised side-effect.

D True
Phenytoin may cause acne and other dermatological side-effects such as coarse facies, dermatological eruptions, and hirsutism. It can also lead to side-effects that affect the gums (see answer to **E** below). It is for these reasons that the *British National Formulary* recommends that phenytoin may be particularly undesirable as a treatment for adolescent patients.

E True
Gingival hypertrophy and tenderness are recognised side-effects.

Question 3.8

Drugs that are effective in the treatment of mania include:

A diazepam

B lithium carbonate

C haloperidol

D promazine

E imipramine.

Answer 3.8

A False
Diazepam is a benzodiazepine with a relatively sustained action that is used short-term for the relief of anxiety or insomnia, and as an adjunct in acute withdrawal from alcohol. It is also used in the treatment of epilepsy and muscle spasm, and in addition has a perioperative use. It is not effective in the treatment of mania.

B True
Lithium carbonate is effective in both the treatment and the prophylaxis of mania. In the treatment of mania the therapeutic response to lithium carbonate usually only occurs after a week. This is a longer response time than is usually the case with antipsychotic drugs such as haloperidol.

C True
The butyrophenone haloperidol is usually effective in bringing the features of acute mania under rapid control.

D False
Although chlorpromazine, a phenothiazine with an aliphatic side-chain, is usually effective in the treatment of mania, the related drug promazine, which is also a phenothiazine with an aliphatic side-chain, is not sufficiently active to be used similarly. Promazine may, however, be of value in the treatment of minor psychiatric problems in the elderly, for example agitation. Another indication is symptomatic relief in terminal illness.

E False
Imipramine is one of the tricyclic antidepressants that is relatively less sedating. It may lead to a worsening of manic symptomatology, and has been reported to occasionally precipitate a manic episode in patients with a bipolar mood disorder.

Question 3.9

The following drugs are benzodiazepines:

A maprotiline

B clorazepate

C medazepam

D meprobamate

E clobazam.

Answer 3.9

The benzodiazepine group of drugs includes:

- alprazolam
- bromazepam
- chlordiazepoxide
- clobazam
- clorazepate
- diazepam
- ketazolam
- lorazepam
- medazepam
- oxazepam
- prazepam.

A   False
Maprotiline is an antidepressant with a tetracyclic nucleus that belongs to the chemical class of dibenzo-bicyclo-octadienes.

B   True
Clorazepate is a tranquilliser that exhibits many of the characteristics of the benzodiazepine group. Particular features that distinguish clorazepate from most other benzodiazepines include the fact that following oral administration nordiazepam appears rapidly in the blood, and there is relatively little sedation.

C   True
Like clorazepate above, medazepam is a benzodiazepine that is used short-term in the symptomatic relief of anxiety.

D   False
Meprobamate is a propanediol with anxiolytic properties accompanied by hypnotic effects. It is less effective than the benzodiazepines and more dangerous in overdosage. It is also anticonvulsant.

E   True
Clobazam is a benzodiazepine that is used short-term in the symptomatic relief of anxiety, as for the benzodiazepines mentioned in **B** and **C** above. It should be noted, however, that many psychiatrists recommend that such benzodiazepines should be used with great care, or not at all, in the treatment of symptomatic anxiety, owing to the risk of dependence. Clobazam may also be used as adjunctive therapy in epilepsy.

Question 3.10

Treatment with chlorpromazine is associated with:

A abnormal T-waves on the ECG

B a decrease in the plasma prolactin level

C hypothermia

D failure of ejaculation

E an increased seizure threshold.

Answer 3.10

A True
In addition to T wave changes, other ECG changes caused by chlorpromazine include an increased QT interval and ST depression. Other cardiovascular side-effects include postural hypotension (see **D** below) and cardiac arrhythmias.

B False
Chlorpromazine causes hyperprolactinaemia, which can manifest itself as galactorrhoea, gynaecomastia, and menstrual disturbances.

C True
A disturbance in temperature regulation is a recognised side-effect. Because of this, chlorpromazine should be used with caution in the elderly, particularly in very hot or very cold weather, as there is a risk of hyperthermia or hypothermia, respectively.

D True
Failure of ejaculation is an antiadrenergic effect; postural hypotension (especially in the elderly) is another such side-effect.

E False
There is a reduction in the seizure threshold. Chlorpromazine should therefore be used with caution in epileptics.

Question 3.11

Features of lithium intoxication include:

A weight gain

B fine tremor

C blurred vision

D dysarthria

E megaloblastic anaemia.

Answer 3.11

The important signs of lithium intoxication are:

- Gastrointestinal
  — anorexia
  — diarrhoea
  — vomiting
- Central nervous system
  — blurred vision
  — muscle weakness and twitching
  — lack of co-ordination
  — mild drowsiness and sluggishness progressing to giddiness with ataxia
  — tinnitus
  — dysarthria
  — coarse tremor

At plasma levels above 2 mM: hyperreflexia and hyperextension of limbs, toxic psychoses, convulsions, syncope, oliguria, circulatory failure, coma, death.

A False
Weight gain is a side-effect of lithium, but not of toxicity.

B False
The tremor in lithium toxicity is coarse; a fine tremor can occur as a non-toxic side-effect.

C True
See above.

D True
See above.

E False
Although lithium can cause an increase in circulating leucocytes, megaloblastic anaemia is not a feature of lithium intoxication.

Question 3.12

Drugs that interact dangerously with monoamine oxidase inhibitors include:

A propranolol

B levodopa

C ephedrine nasal drops

D pemoline

E phentermine.

Answer 3.12

At least 14 days should elapse between stopping a monoamine oxidase inhibitor and commencing any of the following drugs which could induce a hypertensive crisis (this is in addition to avoiding any of these drugs while being treated with the monoamine oxidase inhibitor):

- adrenaline
- dexamphetamine
- levodopa
- metaraminol
- noradrenaline
- pemoline

- dextromethorphan
- ephedrine
- phenylephrine
- phenylethylamine
- phenylpropranolamine
- pseudoephedrine

- fluvoxamine
- tricyclic antidepressants

- diethylpropion
- fenfluramine
- mazindol
- phentermine

A   False
Propranolol is a beta-adrenoceptor blocker and does not interact dangerously with monoamine oxidase inhibitors at therapeutic doses.

B to E   True
See above.

Question 3.13

Side-effects of diazepam include:

A dry mouth

B headache

C respiratory stimulation

D ataxia

E urinary retention.

Answer 3.13

The more important side-effects of benzodiazepines include:

- anxiety (probably a rebound effect)
- confusion and ataxia (especially in the elderly)
- drowsiness
- physical dependence
  — withdrawal symptoms include anxiety symptoms, distorted perception, and neurological disturbances
- psychological impairment (with long-term use).

Other side-effects which occur occasionally include:

- changes in libido
- changes in salivation
- hypotension
- rashes
- urinary retention.

Reported side-effects for which there is conflicting evidence include:

- aggression
- cerebral atrophy.

A and **B True**
See above.

C False
Respiratory depression is a side-effect.

D and **E True**
See above.

Question 3.14

Compared with amitriptyline, mianserin is more likely to cause:

A   haematological reactions

B   anticholinergic effects

C   hepatic reactions

D   cardiovascular reactions

E   hypertensive crisis.

Answer 3.14

A True
In the case of mianserin it is recommended that a full blood count be carried out every 4 weeks during the first 3 months of treatment. If the patient develops a sore throat, pyrexia, stomatitis or other signs of infection, treatment with mianserin should be stopped, and a full blood count should be obtained.

B False
There are fewer and milder anticholinergic side-effects with mianserin compared with amitriptyline.

C True
Mianserin is contra-indicated in severe liver disease. Caution is required with both antidepressants in the treatment of patients with hepatic impairment.

D False
There are fewer and milder cardiovascular effects with mianserin compared with amitriptyline. Therefore mianserin, but not amitriptyline, may be considered suitable for the treatment of a depressed patient with a recent cardiac infarction. Nevertheless, care still needs to be exercised in the pharmacotherapy of such a patient. Mianserin also appears to be safer, at therapeutic dosage, than amitriptyline, in the treatment of patients with cardiac insufficiency or even pre-existing cardiac disease, although again care must be taken.

E False
See the answer to Question 3.12.

Question 3.15

Haloperidol differs from chlorpromazine in that:

A   it has no anti-emetic effect

B   it has no anticholinergic effect

C   it has a greater tendency to cause hypotension

D   it is less sedating

E   it is less likely to cause dystonic reactions.

Answer 3.15

A   False
Both neuroleptics have an anti-emetic effect.

B   False
Haloperidol has fewer anticholinergic effects than chlorpromazine.

C   False
Haloperidol is less likely to cause hypotension than chlorpromazine.

D   True
Haloperidol is less sedating than chlorpromazine.

E   False
Extrapyramidal symptoms, particularly dystonic reactions and akathisia, are more frequent with haloperidol, especially in hyperthyroidism.

Question 3.16

Foods to avoid while being treated with a monoamine oxidase inhibitor include:

A pickled herrings

B cottage cheese

C yeast extract

D game

E milk.

Answer 3.16

Severe hypertensive reactions occur if certain drugs (see the answer to Question 3.12) or foods are taken which contain amines, especially tyramine, that may interact with monoamine oxidase inhibitors. Pharmacies and doctors should give patients being treated with monoamine oxidase inhibitors treatment cards listing precautions that need to be taken.

Foods that may interact with monoamine oxidase inhibitors include:

- cheese, *except*
  - cottage cheese
  - cream cheese
- meat and yeast extracts (e.g. Bovril, Marmite, Oxo)
- alcohol (particularly Chianti)
- nonfresh fish, meat, or poultry
- offal
- avocado
- banana skins
- broad bean pods
- caviar
- herring (pickled or smoked).

These foods should be avoided not only during treatment with monoamine oxidase inhibitors but also up to 14 days after ceasing such treatment.

A   True
See above.

B   False
In general, cheese contains a significant amount of amines (especially tyramine) per unit weight so that it should be avoided by patients taking monoamine oxidase inhibitors; this does not apply, however, to cottage cheese or cream cheese.

C and D   True
See above.

E   False
It is safe to drink milk but, as noted above, cheese (cooked or plain) should be avoided (apart from the types mentioned in **B** above).

FURTHER READING

Berrios G E, Dowson J H (editors) 1983 Treatment and management in adult psychiatry. Baillière Tindall, London (Chapters on Anxiolytic Drugs, Antischizophrenic Drugs and Antidepressant Drugs)

British Medical Association and The Pharmaceutical Press 1989 British National Formulary, No. 18. British Medical Association and The Pharmaceutical Press, London

Kaplan H I, Sadock B J (editors) 1989 Comprehensive textbook of psychiatry, 5th edn. Williams and Wilkins, Baltimore (Chapter on Biological Therapies)

Kendell R E, Zealley A K (editors) 1988 Companion to psychiatric studies, 4th edn. Churchill Livingstone, Edinburgh (Chapter on Drug Treatments)

McGuffin P, Shanks M F, Hodgson R J (editors) 1984 The scientific principles of psychopathology. Grune and Stratton, London (Chapter on Neuropharmacology)

Tyrer P (editor) 1982 Drugs in psychiatric practice. Butterworths, London

4. Descriptive psychopathology

Syllabus requirements

The candidate will be expected to have a basic knowledge of the phenomenology of psychiatry.

Question 4.1

Dysmegalopsia is a recognised symptom of:

A olfactory nerve lesions

B temporal lobe lesions

C hyoscine poisoning

D flashback

E retinal oedema.

Answer 4.1

Dysmegalopsia is a disorder of perception in which there are sensory distortions involving changes in spatial form. It occurs in the visual field and includes the following types:

- macropsia, in which objects are seen larger or nearer than is actually the case
- micropsia, in which objects are seen smaller or farther away than is actually the case.

A False
While lesions of the first cranial nerve can affect the sense of smell, neither macropsia nor micropsia are recognised symptoms.

B True
Dysmegalopsia can occur in temporal lobe lesions such as complex partial seizures. The episodes of dysmegalopsia may occur in attacks prior to fits.

C True
Dysmegalopsia can result from poisoning with hyoscine and other belladonna alkaloids that can affect vision such as atropine.

D True
Flashback is an effect of hallucinogens such as lysergic acid diethylamide (LSD). It is known as the posthallucinogen perception disorder in the Third Revised Edition of the American Psychiatric Association's *Diagnostic and Statistical Manual of Mental Disorders* (DSM-III-R). It consists of the spontaneous transient re-experience, following cessation of use of an hallucinogen, of one or more of the same perceptual symptoms that were experienced during intoxication with the hallucinogen. Dysmegalopsia is a common symptom.

E True
Retinal oedema causes visual images to fall on a functionally smaller area of the retina, thus leading to micropsia.

Question 4.2

The following are included in formal thought disorders:

A concrete thinking

B confabulation

C overinclusive thinking

D persecutory delusions

E derailment.

Answer 4.2

Formal thought disorder refers to disorders of conceptual or abstract thinking which occur in schizophrenia and organic brain disorders. Carl Schneider claimed that five features of formal thought disorder could be isolated:

- fusion — separate ideas are merged and interweaved
- omission — sudden interruption in the stream of thought
- derailment — insertion of inappropriate ideas into the stream
- drivelling — the constituents of an idea are muddled together
- substitution — minor thought is substituted for a major one

There have been other important descriptions of formal thought disorder by Bleuler, Cameron, and Goldstein (see Hamilton 1985 and below). The term is not used officially in DSM-III-R, the reason given being that 'the boundaries of the concept are not clear, and there is no consensus as to which disturbances in speech or thought are included in the concept.'

A   True
Concrete thinking refers to a difficulty in forming abstract concepts. Goldstein built his theory of thought disorder around this.

B   False
Confabulation refers to the fabrication of facts or events in response to questions about situations or events that are not recalled because of memory impairment. It differs from lying in that the person is not consciously attempting to deceive (DSM-III-R). It is common in Korsakov's syndrome.

C   True
Overinclusive thinking refers to an inability to maintain the boundaries of a problem and to restrict operations within their correct limits. The patient cannot narrow down the operations of thinking and bring into action the relevant organised attitudes and specific responses (Hamilton 1985). It has been claimed by Cameron that overinclusive thinking is an outstanding feature of formal thought disorder.

D   False
Delusions are disorders of thought content.

E   True
See above.

Question 4.3

The following may be part of normal experience:

A   circumstantiality

B   feelings of depersonalisation

C   audible thoughts

D   hypnopompic hallucinations

E   autoscopy.

Answer 4.3

A   True
Circumstantiality refers to speech that is indirect and delayed in reaching the point because of unnecessary, tedious details and parenthetical remarks. Circumstantial replies or statements may be prolonged for many minutes if the speaker is not interrupted and urged to get to the point (DSM-III-R). It is commonly seen in many people without a mental disorder.

B   True
Depersonalisation is an alteration in the perception or experience of the self so that the feeling of one's own reality is temporarily lost. This is manifested in a sense of self-estrangement or unreality (DSM-III-R). It sometimes occurs in people who do not have a mental disorder and who are experiencing anxiety, stress, or fatigue.

C   False
This is a Schneiderian first rank symptom.

D   True
Hypnopompic hallucinations take place when the person is falling asleep. The corresponding phenomenon occurring when the person is waking up is known as a hypnagogic hallucination. Both phenomena can occur in normal people who are not suffering from a mental disorder.

E   True
Autoscopy is a strange experience in which the patient sees and recognises himself or herself. It can occur in normal people when, for example, they are tired and exhausted.

Question 4.4

A delusional perception is:

A a false perception occurring in the absence of a stimulus

B a first rank symptom of schizophrenia

C a secondary delusion

D the same as Wahnstimmung

E formed secondary to sensory misperception.

Answer 4.4

A delusional perception is a primary delusion arising fully formed secondary to a normal perception which would otherwise be regarded as unrelated and commonplace. For example, a cupboard door being slightly ajar may be interpreted as a sign that the patient is the King of Spain. The term delusional perception is misleading in that the perceptions are not abnormal, but it is the meaning attached to the normal perception that is delusional. It is one of Kurt Schneider's first rank symptoms of schizophrenia.

A   False
This refers to an hallucination.

B   True
See above.

C   False
A delusional perception is a primary delusion. A secondary delusion can be understood as having arisen from a prior morbid experience.

D   False
The German term Wahnstimmung refers to a change of mood preceding the onset of a delusion in which the patient may have a foreboding that something strange and threatening is about to happen. It is usually translated as delusional mood.

E   False
As noted above, a delusional perception arises secondary to a normal perception.

Question 4.5

The following types of hallucination are correctly paired with conditions in which they characteristically occur:

A   alcoholic hallucinosis — auditory hallucination

B   phobic neurosis — visual hallucination

C   narcolepsy — olfactory hallucination

D   cocaine dependence — formication

E   schizophrenia — extracampine hallucination.

Answer 4.5

A True
Alcoholic hallucinosis is a psychiatric disorder associated with
dependence on alcohol. It is characterised by auditory
hallucinations occurring in the setting of clear consciousness.
The auditory hallucinations tend to be distressing to the patient.

B False
Hallucinations are a feature of psychoses but not of neuroses.

C False
Narcolepsy is characterised by attacks of irresistible sleep
occurring during the day. It is often associated with other
features including hypnagogic hallucinations. Olfactory
hallucinations are not a characteristic feature.

D True
Formication is a type of tactile hallucination in which the patient
feels as though insects are crawling just under the skin. It is
sometimes called the cocaine bug and is characteristic of
dependence on cocaine.

E False
An extracampine hallucination is one that occurs outside the
limits of the sensory field. For example, a patient may hear a
voice talking in Cambridge while aware of the fact that he or she
is in London. Another example would be that of a patient seeing
an object outside his or her visual field. Although extracampine
hallucinations can occur in schizophrenia, they are not
characteristic of this condition. Indeed, according to Hamilton
(1985) extracampine hallucinations do not possess diagnostic
significance; they can also occur in organic brain disorders and
as an hypnagogic phenomenon.

Question 4.6

A lady is seen to be maintaining her arm in the same outstretched position without support over the course of 5 minutes. This could be explained by the following:

A catalepsy

B catatonia

C cataplexy

D hypnosis

E flexibilitas cerea.

Answer 4.6

A True
Catalepsy is a phenomenon that can occur in a catatonic patient in which the patient allows himself or herself to be placed in an uncomfortable posture which is then maintained for long periods without apparent discomfort.

B True
See **A** above.

C False
In cataplexy there is a sudden loss of muscle tone and the patient, if standing, may fall. It is often seen in narcolepsy.

D True
Catalepsy can be induced by hypnosis.

E True
Flexibilitas cerea is also known as waxy flexibility and consists of perseveration of posture in which there is a feeling of plastic resistance as the examiner moves parts of the patient's body. In catalepsy, on the other hand, there is perseveration of posture with no resistance to passive movements; however, when the examiner releases the patient's body the relevant muscles causing the body to adopt the abnormal posture are felt to contract. In spite of this distinction, flexibilitas cerea (or waxy flexibility) is often used synonymously with catalepsy.

Question 4.7

The following are forms of loosening of associations:

A pareidolia

B ambitendence

C verbigeration

D Knight's move

E Vorbeireden.

Answer 4.7

In DSM-III-R loosening of associations is defined as follows:

> Thinking characterized by speech in which ideas shift from one subject to another that is completely unrelated or only obliquely related to the first without the speaker's showing any awareness that the topics are unconnected ... When loosening of associations is severe, speech may be incoherent. The term is generally not applied when abrupt shifts in topics are associated with a nearly continuous flow of accelerated speech (as in flight of ideas).

Loosening of associations occurs in schizophrenia and mania.

A   False
Pareidolia is a disorder of perception in which vivid illusions occur without any conscious effort on the part of the patient. For example, vivid images may be seen in the clouds.

B   False
Ambitendence is a motor symptom in which the patient alternates between two alternate movements.

C   True
Verbigeration is also known as word salad and occurs in the severest form of loosening of associations with utterances being jumbled.

D   True
In Knight's move or derailment there is an inter-sentence or mid-sentence transition from one topic to another. The connection between the two topics is neither logical nor of the type seen in flight of ideas.

E   True
Vorbeireden is a German term that is known in English as talking past the point. 'In this disorder the content of the patient's replies to questions shows that he understands what has been asked and is deliberately talking about an associated topic. For example if asked, "What is the colour of grass?" the patient may reply, "White" ...' (Hamilton 1985).

Question 4.8

Echolalia is observed in:

A schizophrenia

B mental handicap

C phobic neurosis

D idiopathic hypersomnolence

E dementia.

Answer 4.8

Echolalia refers to the repetition of the speech of others. It tends to be persistent and repetitive.

A True
Echolalia may be a feature of catatonic schizophrenia.

B True
Echolalia is seen in such causes of mental handicap as infantile autism.

C False
Echolalia is not a feature of the neuroses.

D False
In idiopathic hypersomnolence the patient complains that he or she is unable to awaken completely for several hours after getting up. Echolalia is not a feature.

E True
Echolalia is seen in dementia.

Question 4.9

Delusions:

A imply the presence of an organic psychiatric disorder

B may be true

C are in keeping with the patient's social and cultural background

D are the product of internal morbid processes

E are unamenable to reason.

Answer 4.9

DSM-III-R defines a delusion as:

> A false personal belief based on incorrect inference about external reality and firmly sustained in spite of what almost everyone else believes and in spite of what constitutes incontrovertible and obvious proof or evidence to the contrary. The belief is not one ordinarily accepted by other members of the person's culture or subculture (i.e., it is not an article of religious faith).

A   False
Delusions can occur in a number of functional psychiatric disorders such as schizophrenia and depressive illness, and so do not imply the presence of an organic psychiatric disorder.

B   True
Although delusions are usually false this is not necessarily always so. For example in some cases of morbid jealousy it may in fact be true that the spouse or partner of the patient is being unfaithful. It is not the truth or otherwise of the delusional belief that is its essential quality; rather it is the fact that a delusion is based on an incorrect inference about external reality that is important.

C   False
Delusions are out of keeping with the patient's social and cultural background.

D   True
It is the fact that delusions are the product of internal morbid processes that makes them unamenable to external influences.

E   True
See above.

Question 4.10

Symptoms of anxiety neurosis include:

A chest pain

B paraesthesiae

C palpitations

D urinary urgency

E hyperreflexia.

Answer 4.10

All true
There are a large number of peripheral manifestations of anxiety neurosis including, for example, diarrhoea, dizziness, hypernydrosis, hyperreflexia, hypertension, palpitations, pupillary mydriasis, restlessness, syncope, tachycardia, tremor, upset stomach ('butterflies'), and urinary frequency, hesitancy and urgency.

The causes of the symptoms can be divided into three major groups:

- autonomic overactivity (e.g. diarrhoea and palpitations)
- overbreathing (e.g. dizziness and paraesthesiae)
- increased muscular tension (e.g. headache and chest pain).

Question 4.11

The following phenomena are illusions:

A phonemes

B the illusion of doubles

C Gedankenlautwerden

D phantom mirror-image

E pareidolia.

Answer 4.11

Illusions are misperceptions of real external stimuli. Although they are more common when the level of consciousness is lowered, they can occur in clear consciousness in the absence of psychiatric disorder.

A False
Phoneme is a term sometimes used in psychiatry to refer to an hallucinatory voice.

B False
In spite of its name, the illusion of doubles, also known as the Capgras syndrome, is not a type of illusion, but a form of delusional misrepresentation in which the patient believes that a closely related person has been replaced by a double.

C False
Gedankenlautwerden is a German term that refers to a type of auditory hallucination in which the voice appears to utter the thoughts of the patient as he or she is thinking them.

D False
The phantom mirror-image is an alternative name for autoscopy and constitutes a special form of hallucination in which the patient sees and recognises himself or herself. See also the answer to Question 4.3**E**.

E True
Pareidolia is a special type of illusion in which vivid illusions occur without any conscious effort on the part of the patient (see also the answer to Question 4.7**A**).

Question 4.12

Dissociation of affect is characteristically seen in:

A   apathy

B   la belle indifférence

C   violent criminals

D   the denial of anxiety

E   alcohol dependence.

Answer 4.12

Dissociation of affect refers to an abnormal expression of emotion in which there is a lack of manifestation of anxiety or fear under conditions where this would be expected.

A False
Dissociation of affect should not be applied to apathy which is strictly speaking a loss of all feeling (Hamilton 1985).

B True
The belle indifférence is a French term that is used to refer to the situation when a conversion hysteric shows less than the expected amount of distress.

C False
According to Hamilton (1985), 'Dissociation of affect should not be applied to the emotional indifference that is often found in violent criminals... It may be that they were callous to begin with, but in any case human beings can become used to anything'.

D True
This is a common situation and may be seen, for example, in soldiers about to enter battle.

E False
In alcohol dependence the patient can be thought of as engaging in the swallowing of affect.

Question 4.13

The following are types of compulsion:

A satyriasis

B dipsomania

C somnambulism

D logorrhoea

E trichotillomania.

Answer 4.13

Compulsions are repetitive and stereotyped seemingly purposeful behaviour patterns. They are also known as compulsive rituals. Compulsions are sometimes labelled as obsessions but strictly speaking compulsions are the motor component of obsessional thoughts.

A   True
Satyriasis is the compulsive need to engage in coitus in the male.

B   True
Dipsomania is the compulsion to drink.

C   False
Somnambulism refers to the phenomenon whereby a complex sequence of behaviours is carried out by a person who rises from sleep and is not fully aware of his or her surroundings at the time.

D   False
Logorrhoea is also known as volubility and refers to speech that is fluent and rambling with many words.

E   True
Trichotillomania is the compulsion to pull out one's hair.

Question 4.14

The following motor disorders are correctly paired with the descriptions given:

A athetosis — random jerky movements

B automatic obedience — pathological automatic imitation of another person's movements

C mannerisms — sudden involuntary irregular movements of small groups of muscles

D stereotypies — repeated involuntary movements that appear to be goal directed

E negativism — motiveless resistance to attempts to be moved.

Answer 4.14

A   False
Athetosis refers to movements that are slow, twisting and writhing. In chorea the movements are abrupt, random, jerky and semi-purposeful.

B   False
In automatic obedience the patient carries out every instruction regardless of the consequences. Echopraxia consists of the pathological automatic imitation of another person's movements, and occurs even when the patient is asked not to continue imitating.

C   False
Mannerisms are repeated involuntary movements that appear to be goal directed. Tics consist of sudden involuntary repeated irregular movements of small groups of muscles.

D   False
Stereotypies consist of repeated regular fixed patterns of movement (or speech) which are not goal directed. The description given is that of mannerisms.

E   True
Negativism consists of motiveless resistance to instructions and to attempts to be moved.

Question 4.15

Complex visual hallucinations occur in the following conditions:

A narcolepsy

B schizophrenia

C centrencephalic epilepsy

D amphetamine psychosis

E occipital lobe tumour.

Answer 4.15

Visual hallucinations are complex when they involve formed images; for example seeing faces or scenes. They are elementary when they involve unformed images; for example seeing flashes of light.

A False
Complex visual hallucinations are not a feature of narcolepsy. The hallucinations associated with this condition are typically hypnagogic ones.

B True
Visual hallucinations are less common than auditory hallucinations in schizophrenia.

C False
Centrencephalic epilepsy is a form of generalised epilepsy that originates in subcortical structures. Complex visual hallucinations are not a feature of centrencephalic epilepsy, but are a feature of complex partial seizures of the temporal lobe.

D True
A paranoid psychosis that cannot be distinguished clinically from acute paranoid schizophrenia may occur in amphetamine psychosis. In addition to complex visual hallucinations, other features include persecutory delusions and auditory hallucinations.

E False
Occipital lobe tumours can give rise to visual hallucinations that are simple, not complex.

Question 4.16

The following types of illusion are recognised features of schizophrenia:

A Fregoli's illusion

B illusion de sosies

C Wahnstimmung

D folie à deux

E Capgras syndrome.

Answer 4.16

All false
A to **E** are all concerned with delusional phenomena; none are illusions.

A
Fregoli's illusion is a condition in which the patient recognises a number of different people as differing in appearance, but has the delusional belief that all of them are in fact the same familiar person (usually a persecutor).

B
Illusion de sosies is the French term by which the illusion of doubles is sometimes known. It is also sometimes known as the Capgras syndrome as mentioned above in the answer to Question 4.11**B**. It is a form of delusional misrepresentation in which the patient believes that a closely related person has been replaced by a double.

C
Wahnstimmung is the German term that is usually translated as delusional mood.

D
Folie a deux is an alternative term for shared delusion. In this condition a person living with a deluded person, usually somebody with whom there is a close relationship, comes to share that person's delusional belief(s).

E
Capgras syndrome — see above.

FURTHER READING

American Psychiatric Association 1987 Diagnostic and statistical manual
of mental disorders, 3rd edn — revised (DSM-III-R). American
Psychiatric Association, Washington DC

Berrios G E 1984 Descriptive psychopathology: conceptual and historical
aspects. Psychological Medicine 14: 303

Gelder M, Gath D, Mayou R 1989 Oxford textbook of psychiatry, 2nd
edn. Oxford University Press, Oxford (Especially the chapters on Signs
and Symptoms of Mental Disorder; and Interviewing, Clinical
Examination, and Record Keeping)

Hamilton M (editor) 1985 Fish's clinical psychopathology, 2nd edn.
Wright, Bristol

Kaplan H I, Sadock B J (editors) 1989 Comprehensive textbook of
psychiatry, 5th edn. Williams and Wilkins, Baltimore (Chapter on
Clinical Manifestation of Psychiatric Disorders)

Kendell R E, Zealley A K (editors) 1988 Companion to psychiatric studies,
4th edn. Churchill Livingstone, Edinburgh (Especially the chapters on
Diagnosis and Classification; and Dependence on Alcohol and Other
Drugs)

Morgan H G, Morgan M H 1989 Aids to psychiatry, 3rd edn. Churchill
Livingstone, Edinburgh (Especially the chapter on Psychopathology)

Sims A C P 1985 Symptoms in the mind. Ballière Tindall, London

5. Explanatory psychopathology

Syllabus requirements

The candidate will be expected to have an awareness of the internal (personality and developmental) and external (environmental) influences which can cause and shape psychopathological phenomena.

Question 5.1

In psychoanalytic theory, the unconscious:

A   contains internal objects

B   is timeless

C   is full of resistance

D   contains childhood wishes that have become fixated

E   tests reality.

Answer 5.1

According to psychoanalytic theory, characteristics of primary process thinking, which occurs in the unconscious, include:

Timelessness
—   the concept of time only develops after a period, in the mind of a child, in connection with conscious reality, e.g. periodicity or chaos of feeding.
Disregard of reality of the conscious world.
Psychical reality
—   memories of a real event and of imagined experience are not distinguished;
—   abstract symbols are treated concretely (as in schizophrenia).
Absence of contradiction
—   opposites have a psychic equivalence; big and small are the same as far as unconsciousness is concerned.
Absence of negation
—   e.g. 'I remember being beaten by a man who was not like my father', may refer to a repressed memory of being beaten by father.

The severance of unconsciousness and consciousness characterises a condition of illness. The basic tenet is that behaviour and subjective experience can have unconscious determinants and this applies to normal and abnormal mental functioning. A large part of the mental apparatus functions outside conscious experience. Ideas and feelings can be regarded as existing unconsciously in one form or another.

A   True

B   True

C   False
Resistance is the name given to everything in words and actions that obstructs access to the unconscious.

D   True

E   False
Reality testing is a process postulated by Sigmund Freud to distinguish stimuli originating in the outside world from the internal world, and to forestall possible confusion between what one perceives and what is only imagined.

Question 5.2

The following concepts are involved in dream work:

A displacement

B death instinct

C hysteria

D condensation

E transitional object.

Answer 5.2

The study of symptom formation and the analysis of dreams led Sigmund Freud to recognise a type of mental functioning that was very different from the thought processes which had been the object of traditional psychological observation. Take for example dreaming. Classical psychology has asserted that dreams were characterised by their absence of meaning. Freud maintained they exhibited a constant sliding of meaning, the mechanisms of which are (1) *displacement*, where an apparently insignificant idea comes to be invested with all the psychical depth of meaning and intensity originally attributed to another one, and (2) *condensation*, a process which enables all the meanings and several chains of association to converge on a single idea standing at their point of intersection, e.g. the overdetermination of a symptom.

A True

B False
The death instinct is the name given, in Freud's final theory of instincts, to that which opposes the life instinct, to bring the living being back to the inorganic state.

C False
Hysteria is a class of neuroses presenting a great diversity of clinical pictures; e.g. *conversion hysteria* in which psychic conflict is expressed symbolically in somatic symptoms (such as hysterical paralysis).

D True

E False
The transitional object is a term introduced by D. W. Winnicott to describe a material object with special value for the baby and young child, that is held, felt, suckled and smelt. It represents both the baby and the mother, until reality testing enables the baby to separate self from other with less anxiety, moving to more mature relationships.

Question 5.3

The following are examples of defence mechanisms:

A repression

B reaction formation

C free association

D narcissism

E sublimation.

Answer 5.3

In psychoanalytic theory, defence mechanisms are special mechanisms to protect consciousness by bringing about a form of dissociation of the energy and ideas from consciousness. Defences by their operation may or may not denote pathology.

A   True
Repression is the basic defence. It is the pushing away of unacceptable ideas and emotions and relegating them to the unconscious. If it is successful no trace of the distressing idea or feeling remains in consciousness but a quantity of affective excitation remains. For example, a person may have forgotten and be unable to recall something which had been read (and which normally it should be possible to remember) because the content of the particular passage aroused unpalatable memories of past sexual events. These memories and emotions would have given rise to the affective reaction of repugnance; the memories, affects, and associated contents of what was read being 'pushed away' from consciousness, i.e. repressed.

B   True
In reaction formation the psychological attitude is diametrically opposed to an oppressed wish and is constituted as a reaction against it. For example, bashfulness may occur to counter exhibitionist tendencies. It is often seen in obsessional character traits.

C   False
Free association is a method employed in psychotherapy in which voice is given without exception to all thoughts which enter the mind.

D   False
Narcissism is a description given originally to account for object choice in homosexuals. It now describes a character type and his or her relationships to others, with love directed towards the image of oneself (as in the myth of Narcissus).

E   True
Sublimation is a process to account for human activities which have no apparent connection with sexuality but which are assumed to be motivated with the force of a sexual instinct, e.g. artistic creation and intellectual enquiry (knowledge to know and ascertain how a baby is made).

Question 5.4

The following statements are true in relation to the transference:

A   It was initially understood by Freud

B   For those involved the transference process remains unconscious

C   It can appear as a passionate demand for love

D   It is the negation of countertransference

E   It can be found in every doctor–patient relationship.

Answer 5.4

The transference is the process in which the patient transfers to the therapist feelings, emotions, and attitudes that were experienced in the patient's childhood in relation usually to his or her parents.

A   True
The transference process was initially understood by Sigmund Freud supervising his colleague Josef Breuer's treatment of an hysterical young woman.

B   True
The substance is conscious whereas the latent content is unconscious.

C   True
Loving as well as negative feelings that are related to affects from the patient's past that, being projected onto the therapist, more easily allow their conscious elucidation.

D   False
The countertransference describes the affect in the therapist that the patient evokes which is not related to the therapist's own particular life. It is an unconscious communication from the patient enabling the therapist to experience what it may have been like being the patient or being in a relationship to the patient at an earlier time.

E   True
Patients will invariably unconsciously place their doctor in a parental position vis-à-vis them as a child.

Question 5.5

In psychoanalytic theory, the transitional object:

A is a term introduced by Ernest Jones

B designates the material object with a special value for the suckling and young child particularly when about to fall to sleep

C is often a teddy bear

D is a me-not me object

E should be kept clean by the mother.

Answer 5.5

A False
The term was introduced by D. W. Winnicott who was a paediatrician and psychoanalyst.

B True

C False
It is the qualities of touch and smell that are important to the infant not its apparent designation by the adult. Thus a whole variety of toys, pillows, and blankets are made use of in this fashion.

D True
This is a part of the transition from the first oral relationship with the mother to a relationship which is much more broadly based. Thus it represents the child's own self and the mother's breast at different times and is used as a period of experimentation.

E False
The smell of it is particularly important to the infant and this can be altered by cleaning, much to the child's anger.

Question 5.6

In psychoanalytic theory, the ego:

A   aims at immediate gratification of needs

B   is only partly conscious

C   is responsible for bringing the defence mechanisms into play

D   identifies with the aggressor

E   is similar to the imago.

Answer 5.6

In psychoanalytic theory it is postulated that development of the mental apparatus leads to the development of the ego and that this is consciousness plus that part of the ego that performs the defence. In other words part of the ego is responsible for bringing the defence mechanisms into play.

A False
It is an aim deriving from the id to have immediate gratification of needs.

B True
Part of it is unconscious like the id, out of which it has evolved.

C True
See above.

D False
This is a mechanism of defence of the ego described by Anna Freud (1936).

E False
The concept of imago is attributed to Carl Jung and des ribes family images of the relationship between the child and its social and family environment.

Question 5.7

A child separated from its mother may pass through the following phases:

A   individuation

B   protest

C   delirium

D   detachment

E   despair.

Answer 5.7

Studies by Bowlby and others have demonstrated that when a child is separated from its attachment figure (usually mother) for at least a few days, then the child may pass through the following phases:

- Protest — e.g. crying
- Despair — apathetic and miserable
- Detachment — the child now seems content and is indifferent to the attachment figure on her return.

A   False
Individuation is a concept of Margaret Mahler as a particular developmental phase in infancy. It is characterised by the child perceiving itself as a separate individual, distinct from its mother.

The concept of individuation also occurs in Jungian theory, and describes the ultimate aim of Jungian therapy. It refers to a continuous life-long process whereby a person comes to have an understanding of their own individuality.

B   True
See above.

C   False
Delirium refers to a confusional state in which the patient is bewildered, disoriented, and restless. It may be associated with fear and hallucinations.

D and E   True
See above.

Question 5.8

In psychoanalytic theory, the following are true of the superego:

A its functions include conscience, self-observation, and the formation of ideals

B it develops out of the perception a person has of the strictures placed by parents and teachers on him or her while growing up

C some patients may be much stricter with themselves (i.e. have a stricter superego) than how their parents used to treat them in reality

D delusions of being watched can be understood in terms of that person's superego

E it appears as an agency embodying law and prohibiting its transgression.

Answer 5.8

All true

A The psychic functions of the superego can be manifested as conscience and self-criticism. Its critical function can lead to the sense of guilt.

B The patient's phantasy of how they were treated by parents may be a gross embellishment of the reality.

C For instance the 'severity' of a person's superego may be inversely proportional to that of the parent.

E But it also contains the desire to be like the good and/or ideal aspect of others.

Question 5.9

Features of normal grief include:

A hallucinations

B loss of appetite

C idealisation of the deceased

D phobic avoidance

E mummification.

Answer 5.9

The features of normal grief, also known as typical or uncomplicated grief, bear a similarity to depressive symptomatology. This was used by Sigmund Freud in his formulation of a theory on the aetiology of melancholia in *Mourning and Melancholia* (1917).

Three stages typically occur:

1. A feeling of numbness and unreality.
2. Symptoms similar to those of depressive disorders, e.g. sadness, loss of appetite, tearfulness, poor concentration, etc.
3. Gradual acceptance.

A   True
In a study by Clayton (1979) brief hallucinations were reported by approximately 10% of bereaved people.

B   True
See above.

C   True
Idealisation of the deceased person is a recognised feature of normal grief.

D   False
Phobic avoidance may be related to excessively delayed grief. Extreme guilt and anger may also occur in such atypical or complicated grief.

E   True
Mummification refers to a behavioural change whereby the bereaved person may try to preserve the belongings of the deceased. It is a feature of normal grief.

Question 5.10

According to Freud's theory of psychosexual development fixation at the anal phase is related in adulthood to:

A generosity

B obstinacy

C obsessionality

D homosexuality

E encopresis.

Answer 5.10

According to Freud's theory of psychosexual development the anal phase occurs between the ages of 1 and 3 years. It is the second phase of psychosexual development in which the anal area and the anal functions of excretion and retention are of importance to the child. Freud proposed that fixation at or regression to this phase can lead to obsessional symptoms and related traits such as parsimony, obstinacy, and orderliness.

In contemporary psychoanalytic theory there has been a movement beyond Freud's psychosexual developmental theory to a greater emphasis on the relationships that occur during development between the child and other people. Important advances in this area have been made by Melanie Klein, Donald Winnicott, Erik Erikson, and Margaret Mahler.

A False

B and **C True**

D False

E False

Encopresis refers to the voluntary or involuntary passage of faeces into inappropriate places (such as clothing or the floor) after the age at which bowel control is usual, in the absence of known organicity.

Question 5.11

The following statements in relation to defence mechanisms are true:

A defence mechanisms are a symptom of a person's illness

B identification with the aggressor was postulated by Anna Freud

C Melanie Klein thought that splitting of the object was a very primitive defence

D psychotics rarely have defence mechanisms

E the particular defence mechanisms a patient uses exert a major influence on when and whether help is sought for a particular symptom.

Answer 5.11

A   False
This statement is not necessarily true as everybody has psychological defences and as such they are necessary for ordinary living in a community and family. Symptoms are *derived* from the final common pathway of the various defence mechanisms available to and used by a person.

B   True
Published in 1936 in her book *The Ego and the Mechanisms of Defence.*

C   True

D   False
Psychotics have more primitive defences such as splitting of the object and what Kleinians call projective identification.

E   True.

Question 5.12

A psychodynamic understanding of depression may include the following:

A psychosomatic reactions such as chest pain

B hyperactive elevated mood

C unresolved mourning for a stillbirth 15 years earlier

D death instinct

E resistance.

Answer 5.12

A, B and **C   True**
A hyperactive elevated mood may constitute a manic defence against depression. Statements **A** and **C** are self-explanatory.

D   False
In the framework of the final Freudian theory of the instincts the death instinct is the name given to the instinct opposed to life with the goal of returning matter to its inorganic state.

E   False
Resistance is the name given to everything in word and action of the analysand that obstructs his gaining access to his unconscious.

Question 5.13

From a psychodynamic perspective features of anxiety neurosis include:

A an expectation of attacks of anxiety

B it is often related to specific traumatic events

C it is usually conscious in the patient's mind

D somatic equivalents

E it is associated with a particular family romance.

Answer 5.13

A and **B**   **True**

C   **False**
The behavioural activity of anxiety is conscious but its deeper structural roots are unconscious.

D   **True**
For example fear of having a heart attack in the absence of organic pathology. The fear of having a heart attack may actually be a wish out of guilt for some thought or action that the person has undertaken which is then somatised.

E   **False**
Family romance is a term for phantasies in which the person imagines his relationship to his parents as being modified such that he is really a changeling and ought really to be a prince. Such phantasies are grounded in the Oedipus Complex.

Question 5.14

The repeated forced rape of a young woman over a weekend by a man who kidnapped her takes place. The following are true:

A it may lead to the woman identifying with the aggressor

B it may lead to a traumatic silence on the part of the victim

C if left unworked through it may lead to the development of a depressive personality with sexual phobias

D if left unworked through it may naturally heal without ill-effect

E it can be postulated that the victimiser was once a victim himself when a child.

Answer 5.14

A True
The defence mechanism of identification with the aggressor enables the woman to split off from her psychic pain and instead causes her to want to find a victim herself instead of being one.

B True
This would be part of a closing off from the emotional impact of the trauma being re-experienced in the telling to another.

C True
This may indeed occur.

D False
This would be analogous to pus being left behind to fester. It is likely to have a grave impairment on future relationships with men, affecting sexual life, marriage, and the rearing of children subsequent to the trauma.

E True
Many rapists have been sexually and physically abused when children, so the cycle of deprivation continues.

Question 5.15

According to conditioning learning theory phobias may result from:

A   extinction

B   classical conditioning

C   isolation

D   primary reward conditioning

E   adventitious reinforcement.

Answer 5.15

A False
Extinction is the gradual disappearance of a conditioned response and occurs when the conditioned stimulus is repeated without the unconditioned stimulus. Experiments have demonstrated that extinction does not entail the complete loss of the conditioned response. Following extinction, if an experimental animal is allowed to rest, a weaker conditioned response re-emerges; this is known as partial recovery.

B True
The American psychologist John Watson (1920) produced a phobia experimentally, using classical conditioning, in an 11-month-old boy known as Little Albert. Before the experiment, Little Albert did not fear white rats. However, following several episodes of pairing in which the presentation of a white rat was accompanied by a loud noise, the boy developed a fear of the rat in the absence of the frightening noise. This was then repeated with a rabbit, and then generalized to any furry mammal. In the development of phobias in general it has been suggested that similar learned responses are of aetiological significance.

C False
Isolation, a defence mechanism, is a concept of psychoanalytic theory not of conditioning learning theory. In psychoanalytic theory it is proposed that a phobia can represent another source of anxiety that has been repressed or displaced.

D False
In primary reward conditioning, which is a type of operant conditioning, a learned response leads to a reward. For example, an experimental animal may receive food or water.

E True
Adventitious reinforcement refers to responses that are accidentally reinforced. It has been suggested in conditioning learning theory that such coincidental pairing of response and reinforcement may lead to the development of a phobia.

Question 5.16

Learning theory concepts implicated in the aetiology of depressive disorders include:

A shaping

B cognitive distortions

C anxiety hierarchy

D acquisition

E learned helplessness.

Answer 5.16

A   False
Shaping refers to the process whereby operant behaviour is changed in a predetermined manner. This is carried out by the selective reinforcement of only those responses that are in the desired direction.

B   True
Cognitive distortions have been put forward by Aaron Beck as an important component of depressive cognitions in cognitive learning theory. Adherents of this theory believe that these cognitive distortions can cause or reinforce depression. Examples of cognitive distortions include magnification and minimisation; arbitary inference; overgeneralisation; and selective abstraction.

C   False
The anxiety hierarchy is a hierarchy of increasing anxiety-evoking stimuli for a given person. It is used in systematic desensitisation.

D   False
The acquisition stage of conditioning is the period during which the association is being acquired between the conditioned stimulus and the unconditioned stimulus with which it is being paired.

E   True
In learned helplessness there is a state of apathy, reduced food intake, and helplessness in laboratory animals which have been exposed experimentally to unavoidable painful stimuli. Seligman suggested that learned helplessness can explain the aetiology of some depressive disorders in humans who feel they are in a hopeless situation over which they have no control.

FURTHER READING

Bowlby J 1973 Attachment and loss, Vol. II. Separation, anxiety and anger. Hogarth Press, London (also Pelican Books 1975)

Clayton P J 1979 The sequellae and non-sequellae of conjugal bereavement. American Journal of Psychiatry 136: 1530–1534

Freud A 1936 The ego and the mechanisms of defence. The Hogarth Press and the Institute of Psycho-Analysis, London

Freud S 1917 Mourning and melancholia. The standard edition of the complete psychological works, Vol. XIV. The Hogarth Press and the Institute of Psycho-Analysis, London

Freud S 1933 New introductory lectures on psycho-analysis. The standard edition of the complete psychological works, Vol. XXII. The Hogarth Press and the Institute of Psycho-Analysis, London

Freud S 1986 The essentials of psychoanalysis. Pelican Books, Harmondsworth

Gelder M, Gath D, Mayou R 1989 Oxford textbook of psychiatry, 2nd edn. Oxford University Press, Oxford (Especially the chapter on Aetiology)

Kaplan H I, Sadock B J (editors) 1989 Comprehensive textbook of psychiatry, 5th edn. Williams and Wilkins, Baltimore (Chapter on Contributions of the Psychological Sciences; also the three chapters on Theories of Personality and Psychopathology)

Kendell R E, Zealley A K (editors) 1988 Companion to psychiatric studies, 4th edn. Churchill Livingstone, Edinburgh (Especially the chapters on Psychology in Relation to Psychiatry; and Personality Development)

McGuffin P, Shanks M F, Hodgson R J (editors) 1984 The scientific principles of psychopathology. Grune and Stratton, London (Chapter on Psychoanalytic Contributions to the Understanding of Psychiatric Illness)

Morgan H G, Morgan M H 1989 Aids to psychiatry, 3rd edn. Churchill Livingstone, Edinburgh

Parkes C M 1985 Review article. Bereavement. British Journal of Psychiatry 146: 11–17

Seligman M E P 1975 Helplessness: on depression, development and death. Freeman, San Francisco

Watson J B, Rayner R 1920 Conditioned emotional reactions. Journal of Experimental Psychology 3: 1–14

Winnicott D W 1953 Transitional objects and transitional phenomena. International Journal of Psychoanalysis 34: 89–97

Wolff H H, Knauss W, Bräutigam W (editors) 1985 First steps in psychotherapy: teaching psychotherapy to medical students and general practitioners. Springer-Verlag, Berlin

6. Clinical assessment and classification

Syllabus requirements

The candidate will be expected to have a basic knowledge of the ways in which psychiatric signs and symptoms are expressed and experienced.

The candidate will be expected to have an understanding of the principles underlying the classification of psychiatric phenomena into syndromes.

Question 6.1

Schneider's first-rank symptoms include:

A   delusions of persecution
B   thought withdrawal
C   voices speaking to the person
D   ideas of reference
E   echolalia.

Answer 6.1

Kurt Schneider's first-rank symptoms of schizophrenia, in the absence of organic disease, were said by him to be of 'special value in helping us to determine the diagnosis of schizophrenia'. However, Schneider made the point that his first-rank symptoms did not always have to be present for such a diagnosis to be made. It should also be borne in mind that they can occur in other functional psychoses, such as mania. The first-rank symptoms are as follows:

thought insertion
thought withdrawal
thought broadcasting
somatic hallucinations
'made' acts/drives/affect
delusional perception
auditory hallucinations
 — audible thoughts
 — voices arguing about subjects
 — voices commenting on actions in the third person.

A   False

B   True

C   False
Second person auditory hallucinations are not a first-rank symptom.

D and **E   False**

Question 6.2

Characteristic features of an obsessional personality include:

A low moral standards

B rigidity in views held

C indecision

D insensitivity to criticism

E unexpressed feelings of resentment.

Answer 6.2

A   False
Moral standards are characteristically high. Indeed a person with this disorder may have a painful guilty preoccupation with thoughts of having 'sinned'.

B   True
A person with an obsessional personality is rigid in his or her views and inflexible in the approach taken to problems.

C   True
There may be a fear of making mistakes, and weighing up the pros and cons of any given new situation may be difficult. This, together with an inhibiting perfectionism, leads to indecision.

D   False
In obsessional personalities sensitivity to criticism is often present.

E   True
Unexpressed feelings of anger and resentment are a common feature, whilst externally little emotion may be displayed. Such angry feelings may be provoked by others interfering with a safe inflexible routine that the person wishes to adhere to. There may also be obsessional thoughts of an aggressive nature.

Question 6.3

Recognised features of agoraphobia include:

A the housebound housewife syndrome
B depersonalisation
C panic attacks
D mania
E obsessional thoughts.

Answer 6.3

Agoraphobia is the commonest type of phobic anxiety neurosis. It is defined in DSM-III-R as 'the fear of being in places or situations from which escape might be difficult (or embarrassing) or in which help might not be available in the event of suddenly developing a symptom(s) that could be incapacitating or extremely embarrassing.' This fear results in the avoidance of agoraphobic situations such as going out alone, public transport, crowds, shops, cinemas, and other public places.

A True
This is the name given to the situation when the agoraphobia is severe enough to cause the patient not to leave home at all.

B True
Depersonalisation was identified as being an important symptom of agoraphobia by Sir Martin Roth (1959). He described the phobic anxiety-depersonalisation syndrome.

C True
It is estimated that at least two-thirds of agoraphobics also have panic attacks. Indeed, in DSM-III-R panic disorder is classified in the following two ways:

- 300.01 Panic Disorder without Agoraphobia
- 300.21 Panic Disorder with Agoraphobia.

Agoraphobia in which there is no evidence of panic disorder is classified in DSM-III-R as:

- 300.22 Agoraphobia without History of Panic Disorder.

D False
Mania is not a recognised feature of agoraphobia. Depression, however, is frequent in this anxiety neurosis.

E True
Obsessional thoughts may occur in agoraphobia.

Question 6.4

Negative symptoms of schizophrenia include:

A disorientation

B auditory hallucinations

C apathy

D emotional blunting

E thought disorder.

Answer 6.4

The distinction between positive or florid symptoms and negative or defect symptoms was originally proposed by the neurologist Hughlings-Jackson in the 19th century. More recently the subtyping of schizophrenia according to whether the symptoms are predominantly positive or predominantly negative has been considered by psychiatrists such as Crow and Andreasen. Negative symptoms include:

- affective flattening
- alogia — e.g. marked poverty of speech, poverty of content of speech
- anhedonia-asociality
- attentional impairment
- avolition-apathy

Negative symptoms tend to be a feature of chronic schizophrenia while positive symptoms are more typical of the acute syndrome.

Andreasen et al have shown that positive symptoms tend to correlate with each other, but that positive symptoms do not correlate with negative symptoms, and *vice versa*. Besides positive and negative schizophrenia, Andreasen and her colleagues have identified a category named mixed schizophrenia in which the patients either do not meet the criteria for positive or negative schizophrenia or else they meet the criteria for both. They have found that in mixed schizophrenia either both negative and positive symptoms are prominent, or neither is prominent.

A   False
Orientation is characteristically normal in chronic schizophrenia. A phenomenon known as age disorientation does, however, sometimes occur in this condition. It refers to the difficulty patients may have in stating their correct age.

B   False
Hallucinations are a positive symptom of schizophrenia. Other positive symptoms include delusions, positive formal thought disorder, and repeated instances of bizarre or disorganised behaviour.

C and D   True
See above.

E   False
See the answer to **B** above.

Question 6.5

Characteristic features of the Ganser syndrome include:

A   hallucinations

B   apparent clouding of consciousness

C   nominal aphasia

D   diurnal variation of mood

E   approximate answers.

Answer 6.5

The Ganser syndrome is an hysterical disorder that was first described in prisoners in the last century. The main features are:

- the giving of approximate answers (e.g. when asked how many legs a cow has, the patient might answer 'five')
- hysterical symptoms
- apparent clouding of consciousness
- hallucinations.

A, B and E   True
See above.

C   False
Nominal aphasia is difficulty in finding the correct name for an object.

D   False
Diurnal variation of mood may be seen in depressive disorders.

Question 6.6

The following, occurring in the absence of an organic disorder, are symptoms of dissociative hysteria:

A amnesia

B aphonia

C paralysis

D somnambulism

E fugue.

Answer 6.6

The hysterical neuroses of the dissociative type are characterised by an apparent dissociation between the normally integrated functions of consciousness, identity, or motor behaviour. In DSM-III-R they are termed the dissociative disorders. The major types in DSM-III-R are:

- 300.12 Psychogenic Amnesia
- 300.13 Psychogenic Fugue
- 300.14 Multiple Personality Disorder
- 300.60 Depersonalization Disorder

Somnambulism also has the essential features of a dissociative disorder, and is classified by DSM-III-R as a Sleep Disorder:

- 307.46 Sleepwalking Disorder.

A True
In psychogenic or hysterical amnesia there is a sudden inability to recall important personal information, the cause not being organic brain disease. Associated features can include perplexity, disorientation, and purposeless wandering.

B and C False
Aphonia and paralysis, not caused by an organic disorder, are symptoms of conversion hysteria. Conversion of symptoms is the mechanism which operates in hysteria where there is a deflection of psychical conflict through somatic symptoms which may be either of a motor nature, e.g. paralysis, or a sensory one, e.g. anaesthesia and pain. The conversion symptoms are typically symbolic of repressed ideas expressed through the medium of the body. Hence the field of psychosomatics.

D True
In somnambulism the patient wakes up, arises, walks around, and may carry out a complex sequence of behaviour, without being conscious of the episode or later remembering it. It usually occurs during slow wave sleep when the patient is not dreaming.

E True
In psychogenic or hysterical fugue there occurs, in the absence of organic brain disease, a sudden unexpected wandering away from one's usual surroundings together with an inability to recall one's former life or identity. There may be associated perplexity and disorientation, and the patient may take on a new identity.

Question 6.7

The following features are more supportive of a diagnosis of cardiac neurosis (irritable heart) than ischaemic heart disease:

A palpitations at rest

B left inframammary pain

C arrhythmia

D history of cigarette smoking

E difficulty in breathing deeply at rest.

Answer 6.7

Cardiac neurosis or irritable heart was described during the American Civil War by da Costa. It is an hypochondriacal disorder in which a patient with normal coronary arteries believes that he or she has heart disease. There is evidence for the involvement of hyperventilation in the production of symptoms seen in this condition, which include palpitations, dyspnoea, fatigue, and left inframammary pain.

A, B and **E   True**
See above.

C   False
Ischaemic heart disease may present as an arrhythmia. More common presentations include a history of cardiac pain (angina of effort) or a history of myocardial infarction.

D   False
Cigarette smoking is associated with an increased risk of coronary atherosclerosis.

Question 6.8

Recognised features of mania include:

A grandiose delusions
B visual hallucinations
C Cotard's syndrome
D delusional perceptions
E unimpaired insight.

Answer 6.8

A   True
Grandiose delusions are often a feature of mania.

B   True
Manic patients may experience 'visions', for example with a religious content.

C   False
Cotard's syndrome is a form of severe depression characterised by extreme nihilistic delusions.

D   True
Schneiderian first-rank symptoms have been reported in about 8–23% of manic patients.

E   False
Although very rarely a patient might consider himself or herself to be ill, full insight is invariably impaired in mania.

Question 6.9

The following motor disorders occur in untreated schizophrenia:

A automatic obedience

B ambivalence

C mitgehen

D forced grasping

E echopraxia.

Answer 6.9

A True
In automatic obedience the patient carries out every command, regardless of the consequences, in spite of having first been told not to do so.

B False
Ambivalence is a type of emotion in which there is the simultaneous presence of opposing impulses towards the same thing. In untreated schizophrenia the motor disorder *ambitendence* may be seen, and refers to alternation between opposite movements.

C True
Mitgehen is an extreme form of co-operation in which the patient will move part or all of the body in the direction of slight pressure on it from the examiner, in spite of having first been told to resist the pressure.

D True
Forced grasping is repeated grasping at another person's outstretched hand, in spite of having first been told not to do so. It is often associated with mitgehen.

E True
Echopraxia is the pathological imitation of another person's movements and occurs even when the patient has been told not to do so.

Question 6.10

In the absence of an organic disorder the presence of the following in a woman would strongly suggest that she is suffering from a psychotic illness:

A obsessional thoughts

B hypnopompic hallucinations

C audible thoughts

D panic attacks

E thought insertion.

Answer 6.10

The term psychotic is defined in DSM-III-R as a 'gross impairment in reality testing and the creation of a new reality.' Perceptions and thoughts are wrongly evaluated, and incorrect inferences are made about external reality. In psychodynamic terms psychosis can be thought of as being a disturbance in the relationship between the ego and the external world.

Features said to occur in psychoses include:

- delusions
- hallucinations
- loss of insight.

A   False
Obsessional disorders are classed as neuroses.

B   False
Although hallucinations are in general a feature of psychoses, hypnopompic and hypnagogic hallucinations often occur as part of normal experience. Thus their presence alone does not strongly suggest a psychotic illness.

C and E   True
These are first-rank symptoms of schizophrenia and in the absence of an organic disorder are strongly suggestive of psychosis.

D   False
Panic attacks occur in anxiety states, which are classed as neuroses.

Question 6.11

Characteristic features of alcoholic hallucinosis include:

A clouding of consciousness

B passivity feelings

C insomnia

D visual hallucinations

E pathological jealousy.

Answer 6.11

All False

Alcoholic hallucinosis is characterised by auditory hallucinations occurring in clear consciousness. The hallucinations may begin as fragmentary sounds, and progress to distressing insults and threats.

Clouding of consciousness and insomnia occur in delirium tremens.

Passivity feelings are not a characteristic feature of alcoholic hallucinosis, although a proportion of chronic cases have been found to develop a schizophrenic picture.

Visual hallucinations occur only infrequently in alcoholic hallucinosis (and are therefore not a characteristic feature), but occur more commonly in delirium tremens.

Pathological jealousy is a complication of alcohol dependence, but is not in itself a characteristic feature of alcoholic hallucinosis.

Question 6.12

Typical symptoms of untreated melancholia include:

A feeling worst in the morning

B increased weight

C creative overactivity

D agitation

E dread of the future.

Answer 6.12

According to Kendell (1988) melancholia 'is known variously as endogenous, endogenomorphic, psychotic, retarded, vital and manic-depressive depression. None of these terms is satisfactory and . . . the old word melancholia . . . is preferable.'
(*Companion to Psychiatric Studies,* 4th edition, page 336.) The DSM-III-R diagnostic criteria for the melancholic type of major depression include:

- anhedonia
- lack of reactivity to stimuli that are usually pleasurable
- depression regularly worse in the morning
- early morning awakening
- psychomotor retardation or agitation
- loss of appetite and weight.

A   True
See above.

B   False
To meet the DSM-III-R criteria the weight loss must be significant, defined as, for example, a loss of more than 5% of the body weight in a month.

C   False
Retardation is typical in melancholia.

D   True
Agitation is common, with the patient typically being restless, pacing aimlessly, plucking at buttons, etc. Agitation may co-exist with retardation; the two are not mutually exclusive.

E   True
Patients are often convinced that they will not recover and that the future is hopeless, with no end in sight to their misery. Hence there is a high risk of suicidal thoughts and subsequent deliberate self harm.

Question 6.13

In neurotic disorders:

A   symptoms may persist even when the original cause has disappeared

B   genetic factors are of little or no importance

C   the death rate is greater than average

D   stressful conditions at work are an important cause

E   medication is an effective form of long-term treatment.

Answer 6.13

Neuroses may be considered to be mental disorders in which reality testing is intact and exaggerated forms of normal reactions to stressful events occur. The symptoms are distressing and unacceptable (ego-dystonic) and, without treatment, are relatively long-lived and recurrent.

In psychodynamic terms neuroses can be thought of as psychogenic manifestations in which the symptoms represent symbolic expressions of psychic conflict. The origins of the latter may lie in childhood history. Such symptoms constitute a compromise between wishes and defences.

A True
This may be seen, for example, in cases of phobia and anxiety states.

B False
Genetic studies indicate that there is a moderate genetic influence in many of the neuroses. For example, a twin study by Slater and Shields (1969) looking at rates of concordance in anxiety neuroses found a concordance rate of approximately 40% in monozygotic pairs and 15% in dizygotic pairs.

C True
The death rate among neurotic patients has been shown to be increased by a factor of 1.5 to 2 among outpatients, and 2 to 3 among inpatients (see Sims 1978).

D True
One of the studies that has indicated that stressful conditions at work can be involved in causing neurotic symptoms is that by Parkes (1982) of student nurses changing from medical to surgical wards. After making this change, the student nurses reported more neurotic symptoms in the wards that they rated as being more stressful and less satisfying to work in.

E False
In general, medication is not an effective form of long-term treatment for neurotic disorders. Social and psychological forms of management, including the psychotherapies, may be helpful.

Question 6.14

The following statements regarding hysteria are correct:

A conversion hysteria has anxiety attached in a more or less stable fashion to a specific external object such as a phobia

B anxiety hysteria is exemplified by the cyclical conflict being expressed symbolically in somatic symptoms of many kinds

C essentially hysteria is 'a malady through representation'

D hysterics use sublimation as a major defence mechanism

E hysterics are preoccupied with screen memories.

Answer 6.14

A False

Conversion hysteria is exemplified by the cyclical conflict being expressed symbolically in somatic symptoms of many kinds.

B False

Anxiety hysteria has anxiety attached in a more or less stable fashion to a specific external object such as a phobia. (The descriptions given in parts **A** and **B** of the question are reversed.)

C True

The quote is after Janet's 1894 description published in *The Mental State of Hystericals*.

D False

Sublimation is a defence mechanism which raises more base desires to a more sublime potential such as the work ethic or art.

E False

Screen memory is a childhood memory characterised both by its sharpness and its apparent insignificance of contents. Its analysis leads back to indelible childhood experiences and unconscious phantasies.

Question 6.15

Characteristic features of Alzheimer's disease include:

A   auditory hallucinations

B   palilalia

C   dressing apraxia

D   ophthalmoplegia

E   disorientation for time and place.

Answer 6.15

A False
Auditory hallucinations are not a characteristic feature of
Alzheimer's disease.

B True
Palilalia is a form of perseveration of speech. The perseverated
word is repeated with increasing frequency.

C True
Dressing apraxia occurs in Alzheimer's disease together with
other features of parietal lobe dysfunction.

D False
Ophthalmoplegia refers to extraocular muscle paresis and
occurs, for example, in Wernicke's encephalopathy, myasthenia
gravis, and progressive supranuclear ophthalmoplegia (the
Steele–Richardson–Olszewski syndrome).

E True
Disorientation for time and place is an important and relatively
early feature of this condition.

Question 6.16

Characteristic features of sociopathic disorder include:

A delusions of grandeur

B crimes of violence are planned

C lack of conscious guilt

D a good response to psychiatric treatment

E inability to form enduring loving relationships.

Answer 6.16

Sociopathic personality disorder is termed antisocial personality disorder in DSM-III-R. There is a pattern of irresponsible and antisocial behaviour starting in childhood or early adolescence, and continuing into adulthood very often in relation to profound early trauma. Characteristic features include:

- failure to learn from adverse experiences
- failure to make loving relationships
- impulsive actions
- lack of guilt.

A False
Delusions of grandeur are not a characteristic feature of this disorder. They are commonly seen, however, in mania (see Question 6.8).

B False
There are often repeated offences against the law. They tend to be impulsive.

C True
There usually is no conscious sense of guilt. Psychodynamically the unconscious guilt is split off and often projected or imposed on others. For example the doctor may feel guilty for his or her difficulty in treating such a patient.

D False
Various types of psychiatric treatment have been tried for sociopathic personality disorder, but in general the response is not good owing to the difficulty of making a treatment alliance.

E True
See above.

FURTHER READING

American Psychiatric Association 1987 Diagnostic and Statistical Manual of Mental Disorders, Third Edition — Revised (DSM-III-R). American Psychiatric Association, Washington D.C.

Andreasen N C, Olsen S 1982 Negative v positive schizophrenia. Archives of General Psychiatry 39: 789–794

Berrios G E 1987 Outcome prediction and treatment response in schizophrenia. Practical Reviews in Psychiatry, Series 2, 3: 7–9

Berrios G E, Dowson J H (editors) 1983 Treatment and management in adult psychiatry. Baillière Tindall, London

Gelder M, Gath D, Mayou R 1989 Oxford textbook of psychiatry, 2nd edn. Oxford University Press, Oxford

Hamilton M (editor) 1985 Fish's clinical psychopathology, 2nd edn. Wright, Bristol

Kaplan H I, Sadock B J (editors) 1989 Comprehensive textbook of psychiatry, 5th edn. Williams and Wilkins, Baltimore

Kendell R E, Zealley A K (editors) 1988 Companion to psychiatric studies, 4th edn. Churchill Livingstone, Edinburgh

Lader M H 1969 Studies of anxiety. British Journal of Psychiatry Special Publication No. 3 (Slater E, Shields J Genetic aspects of anxiety)

Morgan H G, Morgan M H 1989 Aids to psychiatry, 3rd edn. Churchill Livingstone, Edinburgh

Parkes K R 1982 Occupational stress among student nurses: a natural experiment. Journal of Applied Psychology 67: 784–796

Roth M 1959 The phobic anxiety-depersonalization syndrome. Proceedings of the Royal Society of Medicine 52: 587–595

Rubenstein D, Wayne D 1985 Lecture notes on clinical medicine, 3rd edn. Blackwell Scientific, Oxford

Sims A C P 1978 Hypotheses linking neuroses with premature mortality. Psychological Medicine 8: 255–263

Sims A C P 1985 Symptoms in the mind. Baillière Tindall, London

7. The MRCPsych Part I Examination

The MRCPsych Part I examination tests basic clinical psychiatry. Candidates are expected to demonstrate knowledge of the subject, including relevant aspects of basic sciences, and practical skills at the level appropriate on completing 1 year of full time post-registration experience in an approved post. According to the Regulations knowledge of the subject and practical skills are of equal importance in testing the candidate's competence. There is one multiple choice question paper and a clinical examination.

The multiple choice question paper

This paper consists of 50 questions to be answered in $1\frac{1}{2}$ hours. Thus there is an average of 108 seconds available for each question. The syllabus requirements for each subject examined have been given at the beginning of each of the above chapters. It is strongly recommended, however, that the candidate also reads the latest regulations in force at the time of taking the examination.

Each question consists of a stem followed by five items, **A** to **E**. Each of these items may be true (*T*) or false (*F*). All the items in a question may be true, and all may be false. One mark is gained (+1) for every item correctly completed. One mark is lost (-1) for each item incorrectly completed. For each item not answered a mark is neither gained nor lost (0).

Since marks are lost for incorrect answers, it is the view of the authors that guessing answers at random is *not* to be recommended. (One book for this examination actually recommends a system of adding up the total number of *Ts* and *Fs* and then using this to work out whether remaining unanswered items in a question are true or false. This is an extremely dangerous 'method' which can result in the loss of many valuable marks.)

It is recommended that candidates arrive well in time for both parts of the examination. For the multiple choice question paper it is often the case that candidates have to be sitting at their desks 10 minutes or so before the official starting time. It is also important to keep a close watch on the time during the examination.

The clinical examination

The candidate will be expected to have the requisite knowledge about practical procedures. Thus he or she will be required to understand the principles underlying the clinical methods of psychiatry: the establishing of a satisfactory working relationship with the patient, the eliciting of accurate information under the several headings of the psychiatric history, the procedures for examining the patient's mental state and related abnormalities on physical examination, and the integrating of this information in clinical assessment with recognition of the need for further examination, information and/or investigations. A detailed plan of management is not required. (The latter is tested in the Part II Examination.)

In the MRCPsych Part I Examination, the clinical examination must be passed in order to pass the whole examination. A good pass in this part of the examination may be sufficient to allow a candidate who has narrowly failed in the multiple choice paper to pass overall. However, the converse is not true, i.e. however well a candidate does on the multiple choice paper, failing the clinical examination will result in failure of the whole MRCPsych Part I Examination.

Candidates will be expected to examine a case or cases which may be drawn from any aspect of adult general psychiatry for 50 minutes. During the 30 minute interview with a pair of Examiners, candidates are expected to further interview the patient for about 10 minutes in the presence of the Examiners. The main areas of assessment are the candidate's ability to establish a satisfactory relationship with the patient, take a full psychiatric history, carry out an accurate mental state examination, make appropriate deductions from the information available to him or her, and come to a conclusion concerning the diagnosis and differential diagnosis of the disorder(s) from which the patient is suffering.

Candidates will not be expected to carry out a physical examination as a routine, but a selective examination should be undertaken if this seems to be called for by observations made during the interview. These may include examination of the pulse, blood pressure, fundi, extrapyramidal system, etc. The necessary instruments and facilities will be available during the clinical examination.

Further useful details of approaches to the clinical skills required for this part of the examination are to be found in the books listed at the end of this chapter. From the point of view of the clinical examination of MRCPsych Part I in particular, candidates are recommended to read Part Three of *Aids to Psychiatry* by Professor H. G. Morgan, and the chapter that deals with this part of the examination in the authors' sister book of examination notes.

FURTHER READING

Gelder M, Gath D, Mayou R 1989 Oxford textbook of psychiatry, 2nd edn. Oxford University Press, Oxford. (Chapter 2: Interviewing, Clinical Examination, and Record Keeping)

Holden N 1987 Examination technique in psychiatry. Edward Arnold, London

Institute of Psychiatry 1973 Notes on eliciting and recording clinical information. Oxford University Press, Oxford

Kendell R E, Zealley A K (editors) 1988 Companion to Psychiatric Studies, 4th edn. Churchill Livingstone, Edinburgh. (Chapter 10: The Psychiatric Interview)

Leff J P, Isaacs A D 1981 Psychiatric examination in clinical practice. Blackwell Scientific, Oxford

McGuffin P, Greer S 1987 A psychiatric catechism. Edward Arnold, London

Morgan H G, Morgan M H 1989 Aids to Psychiatry, 3rd edn. Churchill Livingstone, Edinburgh. (Part Three: On Taking Examinations)

The Royal College of Psychiatrists 1987 General Information and regulations for the MRCPsych Examinations, 8th revision. The Royal College of Psychiatrists, London

The Royal College of Psychiatrists 1985 Report to the Court of Electors, The Royal College of Psychiatrists Working Party for Review of the MRCPsych. The Royal College of Psychiatrists, London